STUDENTS GO GOURMET

by Sophia Khan and Ellen Bass

DAILEY
Swan
PUBLISHING

Dedication

Dedicated to the city and people of New Orleans. A portion of proceeds will be donated
to sustainable post-hurricane redevelopment efforts in the Ninth Ward.
Look for an original New Orleans tribute recipe in each chapter.

Thanks

We would like to thank our friends and family for their love and support.
A special thank you to our agent Chamein Canton for her steadfast encouragement and untiring faith.

TABLE OF CONTENTS

6. Gourmet Sandwiches and Burgers   80

Thanksgiving Burger
Moroccan Burger with Mint Mayonnaise
Ham and Quattro Formaggi Panino
Crab Cake Burger
Mexican Burger with Mole Sauce
Panino Caprese
New Orleans Oyster Po' Boy Sandwich
Vienna Wiener Dogs
Portabella on a Portuguese Muffin
French Chicken Salad Sandwich

7. Pasta   102

Refreshing Farfalle
Lemon Pasta
Pomegranate Pasta
Gorgonzola Portabella Penne
Spaghetti with Keftethes and Garlic Bread
New Orleans Andouille Pappardelle
Moroccan Stuffed Shells with Curried Béchamel
Artichoke Pesto Alfredo
Cheese Tortellini with Pumpkin and Fried Sage

8. Meat and Fish   122

Garlic Shrimp Orzo
Choco-chili
Salmon Risotto with Caper Cream Sauce
Filet Mignon with Truffled Mashed Potatoes
21st Century Pork Chops and Apple Sauce
Yia-Yia's Chicken Tenders with Homemade Honey Mustard Sauce
New Orleans Shrimp Étouffée
Seared Tuna Tacos
Coconut Pecan Crusted Tilapia with Warm Mango Pineapple Salsa
Seared Bass on Artisanal Pasta
Angel Citrus Salmon

1. THE BARE NECESSITIES

The Basic Necessities:

- Saucepans
- Sauté pans
- Nonstick sauté pan (especially important for making crepes)
- Stock pot
- Baking sheet
- Broiler pan (usually comes with the oven)
- Lasagna dishes
- Colander (for draining pasta and washing veggies)
- Zester/Microplane
- Paring knife
- Serrated knife (knife with teeth--great for slicing tomatoes and bread)
- Santoku knife (great general all-purpose knife)
- Knife sharpener
- Pastry brush
- Cutting board (plastic or wood)
- Measuring cups (wet and dry)
- Measuring spoons
- Can opener
- Small food processor (2 cup)
- Candy thermometer
- Whisk
- Soup Ladle
- Cooking utensils (spatula, wooden spoon, slotted spoon)
- Rolling pin
- Manual citrus juicer
- Mixing bowls
- 1 quart ice cream maker
- Hand-held electric mixer

Advanced Necessities:

- Stand mixer
- Large capacity food processor (8 – 14 cup)
- Complete knife set
- Electric citrus juicer
- Crepe pan
- Risotto pan

2. THE WELL STOCKED STUDENT'S KITCHEN

Spices & Herbs

· Ground Cumin
· Cinnamon
· Ancho chili powder
· Ground thyme
· Saffron threads
· Cayenne pepper
· Onion powder
· Garlic powder
· Dried Oregano
· Kosher salt
· Ground black pepper
· Almond extract
· Vanilla extract
· Fresh herbs (last a week in the refrigerator):
· Thyme
· Tarragon
· Rosemary
· Sage
· Cilantro

Canned Foods

· Olives
· Refried beans
· Chick peas (Garbanzo beans)
· Cannellini beans
· Kidney beans
· Black beans
· Diced tomatoes
· Crushed tomatoes
· Corn
· Artichoke hearts
· Coconut milk
· Tuna

Baking Supplies

· Flour
· Pancake/Waffle mix
· Sugar (white refined)
· Brown sugar
· Sugar cookie mix
· White chocolate morsels
· Milk chocolate morsels
· Oats
· Macadamia nuts
    (once opened, do not keep more than 1 month)
· Pecans (once opened, do not keep more than 1 month)
· Unsalted cashew nuts
· Raw peanuts

General Pantry Items

· Honey
· Chicken stock
· Blueberry preserves
· Fig preserves
· Olive oil
· Vegetable oil
· Sesame oil
· Red wine vinegar
· Champagne vinegar
· Rice wine vinegar
· Balsamic vinegar
· Dried pasta
· Instant grits
· Corn chips
· Hamburger/hot dog rolls
· Pita bread
· Aluminum foil/parchment paper/plastic wrap

Refrigerator Items

- Sour cream
- Mascarpone cheese
- Gorgonzola cheese
- Goat cheese
- Eggs
- Milk
- Half n'Half
- Unsalted Butter
- Shredded cheese
- Grated Parmesan cheese
- Tomato paste in a tube
- Garlic paste in a tube
- Lemon juice in a plastic lemon
- Lime juice in a plastic lime
- Capers
- Mayonnaise
- Tahini (sesame seed paste)
- Wasabi paste
- Hot sauce
- Dijon mustard
- Sweet relish

Freezer Items

- Puff pastry sheets
- Puff pastry cups
- Phyllo dough/cups
- Pre-made Pizza crusts

Fresh Fruits/Vegetables
remember to store your fruits and veggies as they were in the store

- Apples
- Lemons/Limes
- Bananas
- Avocados
- Mangos
- Tomatoes
- Garlic
- Yellow onions
- Shallots
- Mushrooms
- Lettuce

3. Culinary Lingo

Aioli:
A sauce of mayonnaise plus garlic. Other ingredients, such as preserves, herbs, or spices, can be added depending on the flavor palate you want to create. Garlic aioli, for instance, is an unbeatable dipping sauce for French fries, while blueberry preserve aioli is fantastic slathered on a hamburger bun—see our Bar Harbor dinner for details!

Al Dente:
An Italian expression meaning "to the tooth," usually used when referring to pasta that has been cooked 1 – 2 minutes less than package directions and slightly firm to the bite.

Aluminum foil:
An indispensible kitchen item that can be used for wrapping foods for freezing or in a hot oven to line a dish for easy clean up. It can also be used on a grill, especially for fish and other foods that may otherwise fall apart on the hot grill surface. A great way to preserve the internal juices.

Anise:
An herb that imparts a licorice flavor and fragrance, commonly featured in South Asian cuisine.

Antioxidants:
Any substance that promotes health by prevention of the production of free radicals in the body. Free radical cell damage is associated with the development of cancer.
Examples of antioxidants found in foods
- Beta carotene: carrots, sweet potatoes, kale, mangos, apricots, spinach
- Lycopene: tomatoes, watermelon, apricots, guava, papaya
- Vitamin C: in citrus fruits
- Vitamin A: sweet potatoes, carrots, milk, liver, egg yolks
- Vitamin E: almonds, wheat germ, safflower oil, corn oil, soybean oil, mangos, nuts
- Polyphenols: green tea and pomegranate.

Antipasto:
An Italian appetizer assortment typically consisting of smoked meats, cheese, olives, and marinated vegetables.

Appetizer:
The first course of a meal, not to be confused with hors d'oeuvre (which are savory foods that can be served as appetizers or before the meal).

Arrabiatta:
A spicy tomato-based sauce usually served over pasta or fish.

Baba Ganoush:
A dip made with eggplant, tahini, garlic, and lemon juice; +/- tomatoes, onion, parsley, or cumin depending on what part of the world the recipe hails from.

Bake:
To cook food in an oven.

Béarnaise:
A warm sauce made with egg yolks, butter, vinegar, shallots, and tarragon. Named after a city in the Pyrenees, this sauce is wonderful over filet mignon.

Béchamel Sauce:
One of the Mother Sauces of French cuisine, this sauce is made with flour, butter, and milk.

Blanch:
To cook foods in boiling water for only a minute or two to preserve color and crispness. Traditionally, the food is immediately placed in ice water to halt the cooking process and to preserve the color—frequently called "shocking" the food. Asparagus and green beans are often blanched in this manner.

Blind Bake:
To bake a pie shell prior to filling it, as when making a quiche. The filling will cook more quickly than the dough, and the dough will therefore be undercooked if blind baking of the shell does not occur first.

Braise:
Slow cooking in liquid in a covered pot. Osso bucco is a classic example of braised veal shanks.

Broil:
Cooking by direct exposure to high heat. The broiler coils are located on the top inner surface of an even. Fish is wonderful under the broiler lightly covered with aluminum foil. For those of you without a toaster, the broiler is an excellent and easy solution to toasting bread. The broiling process is extremely quick, so watch carefully to make sure your food does not burn.

Buttermilk:
The liquid left over during the process of making butter. Today, it is made from skim milk, to which a culture has been added to produce a thick texture. Buttermilk has a tangy taste and is frequently used in making biscuits and in the batter for fried chicken.

Calamari:
Italian for squid, often found on menus as a fried appetizer. For a healthier alternative, sauté and serve with pasta or salad.

Caper:
A flower bud from a shrub in the Mediterranean and Middle East. This edible bud is delicious with fish, in cream sauces, and in spreads such as tapenade. Since capers are naturally very salty, you will want to reduce (or even eliminate) the salt in your recipe when using them.

Caramelize:
To create a brown crust on food by heating sweet substances such as sugar or the natural sugars in food. Sprinkling sugar atop a custard and placing under the broiler or heating with a kitchen torch makes the firm top of a crème brulee. The natural sugars in pineapple caramelize when placed on a grill, imparting a sweet and crunchy crust.

Caviar:
Fish roe (eggs), an expensive delicacy that truly elevates your meal to gourmet.

Chevre:
The French word for goat, often used to refer to goat cheese.

Chickpea:
Also called a garbanzo bean. A very versatile and healthy bean used in a wide variety of cuisines, especially Middle Eastern staple dishes such as hummus and falafel.

Chiffonade:
From the French meaning "made of rags," chiffonade refers to the process of cutting food into thin ribbons. Usually a technique applied to small leaves (basil, sage) or lettuce. See our instructional DVD for the two proper methods of applying the chiffonade.

Chop:
To cut food into small pieces, in the form of a rough chop, dice, mince, etc.

Cilantro:
A fresh herb used in cuisine worldwide, indispensable to guacamole. Dried cilantro is called coriander and often appears in South Asian dishes.

Compound butter:
Butter mixed with ingredients such as dried or fresh herbs. You can add anything you think will taste good. Butter should be mixed with your ingredient of choice, after which it is rolled in a log and stored in the refrigerator or freezer until reaching desired firmness. Gorgonzola butter is delicious over steak.

Crème brulee:
Baked custard topped with a crunchy layer of caramelized sugar.

Crème fraiche:
The French version of sour cream native to Normandy; thicker and less sour than traditional sour cream.

Cumin:
A spice popular in Indian and Middle Eastern cooking, availablein seed form as well as ground. Cumin adds a smoky, earthy flavor to food. Being particularly potent, only a small amount is necessary to add incredible layers of rich complexity to food.

Custard:
A dish made from a base of milk and eggs. Custards can be sweet, like vanilla bean crème brulee, or savory, like saffron crème brulee. Baked custards, such as saffron crème brulee, are labor intensive. They require slow cooking in a low oven in a water bath to evenness. Custards also serve as the bases for ice cream.

Deglaze:
To create a sauce from pan drippings by adding liquid (such as broth, stock, or wine) after the meat has been removed. The liquid and pan drippings then cook at a slow boil or simmer until thick and ready to coat the cooked meat.

Dice:
To cut food into cube-sized pieces. Dicing creates larger pieces than mincing but is more precise than a rough chop.

Dilute:
To decrease the concentration of a liquid, typically by adding water.

Dredge:
To coat food with a dry ingredient like flour, as in the process of coating raw oysters with batter to make fried oysters.

Edamame:
Japanese for soybeans. Great for healthy snacking and versatile for a range of cuisines.

Encrust:
To form a crust. For example, placing crushed pecans over trout before cooking.

Entrée:
The main course of a meal.

Escargot:
The French name for snail, delicious when cooked in garlic and oil.

Fats:
Fats can be broken down into 2 major categories:
Bad Fats – saturated fats and trans fats
Good fats – monounsaturated fats and polyunsaturated fats

  Examples:
  Bad Fats – saturated fats and trans fats
  · Saturated fats: meats and dairy
  · Trans fats: commercially baked goods and fried foods

  Good fats – monounsaturated fats and polyunsaturated fats
  · Monounsaturated fats: canola oil, olive oil, peanut oil, safflower oil, avocados, nuts, seeds
  · Polyunsaturated fats: soybean oil, safflower oil, oily fish like salmon, tuna, mackerel, herring, and trout

Fennel:
A plant that can be used as an herb, spice, or vegetable. The entire plant is edible and has a subtle licorice flavor, like anise.

Filet Mignon:
A single serving of steak cut from the tenderloin, which is the psoas muscle (a hip flexor) of an animal. Although it tends to be more expensive, the meat is delicious and melts in your mouth when cooked to perfection.

Flan:
Another alias for crème caramel. It is a custard-based dessert with a caramel topping. The caramel is made in the bottom of the ramekin, and the custard is then poured on top. After cooking, flip the dessert upside down and voila, a flan!

Food processor:
A machine invented in France in the 1960s that makes chopping and pureeing foods quick and easy. Most machines can be fitted with different blades corresponding to different settings, such as chop, grate, or julienne. The work bowl of the processor varies from small (2-cup capacity) to large (14cup capacity). The small food processors are readily available at grocery stores and department stores, and they extremely affordable—as well as indispensable to cooking!

Frittata:
A baked omelet, Italian in origin. The omelet is started on the stove but finished under the broiler or baked at 425 degrees F. Popular additions to the frittata include cheese, herbs, meat, and vegetables.

Fry:
To cook food in oil that has been preheated to 350 – 375 degrees F after coating the food in flour or batter.

Heirloom:
Vegetables or fruits that grow by open pollination. Heirloom tomatoes are also known as Ugli tomatoes.

Herb:
A plant used to season food. Herbs are usually the leaves of herbaceous plants, meaning plants that have stems that are fleshy rather than woody. Can be pronounced with or without the silent 'h.' Examples of herbs typically used in cooking are: parsley, basil, tarragon, and rosemary. Herbs can be purchased fresh or dried. You should note, however, that dried herbs are more concentrated than fresh. The substitution ratio for fresh: dried is 3:1.

Hollandaise sauce:
One of the French cuisine Mother Sauces served warm, typically over Eggs Benedict, made with eggs, butter, and lemons.

Hors d'oeuvres:
Dishes that are served before the meal. In French, it means "outside the main work" of the meal. Can be confused with appetizers but really means dishes that are served when guests arrive, such as hummus, gorgonzola bites, smoked salmon on toast points, and others. Both hot and cold, they are excellent with cocktails or aperitifs. The Spanish equivalent is tapas.

Hummus:
A dip or spread made from chickpeas, garlic, lemon, and tahini, a staple of Mediterranean and Middle Eastern cuisines.

Julienne:
To cut a vegetable or citrus rind into thin strips, usually the thickness of a matchstick (and therefore thicker than a chiffonade).

Marinate:
To flavor and tenderize meat or fish by immersing it in a liquid flavoring (marinade) for several hours prior to cooking. Be careful when using an acidic liquid (such as citrus or vinegar) not to marinate fish for more than 1 hour, because the fish will begin to cook! This technique is popular in Spanish cuisine in the dish ceviche.

Mascarpone:
Very rich Italian cream cheese used in both sweet and savory dishes. It is the classic cheese used in tiramisu.

Mayonnaise:
A cold sauce made through an emulsion of eggs, oil, vinegar, salt, and pepper. It is the Mother Sauce of cold sauces.

Melt:
To liquefy a solid by warming it.

Mince:
To chop into very small pieces, smaller than both rough chopping and dicing.

Mis In place:
in French translates roughly to "everything in its place." Refers to having all of your ingredients measured and equipment/pans ready before you begin cooking.

Mother Sauce:
A basic sauce in French cuisine to which diverse ingredients can be added. Examples include hollandaise sauce and mayonnaise.

Onions:
One of the oldest and most widely used vegetables in human cuisine worldwide.
Common Varieties
- Vidalia: a sweet, mild onion that can be eaten like an apple
- Red: also sweet and can be consumed raw, delicious in salads and sandwiches as well as on the grill
- Yellow: the classic cooking union, a bit too sharp for most people to eat raw
- Green: also called scallions, used in finishing a dish such as potato salad and Pad Thai. Popular in Asian cuisine.

Orzo:
Pasta used in Mediterranean cooking that strongly resembles rice grains.

Pancetta:
Salt-cured, spiced pork belly. It is similar to traditional bacon and sometimes referred to as Italian bacon, but unlike bacon is not smoked. Wonderful in creamy pasta sauces and an excellent substitute for bacon in recipes such as salad Lyonnaise.

Panko:
Japanese breadcrumbs, ideal for coating fish, poultry, meat, vegetables, and even tofu.

Parchment paper:
Silicon-treated paper that is used to line pans for non-stick cooking and easy clean up. It does not need to be buttered or oiled and can be used in an oven up to 420 degrees F or in a microwave. Do not put parchment paper in a toaster oven, under the broiler, or in halogen light ovens—this is a fire hazard.

Peppers:
Hot or sweet vegetables common in cuisine the world over, sometimes referred to as chili peppers. The heat in peppers comes from a natural substance called capsaicin, which is measured in Scoville units. Counteracting the heat is accomplished best with milk and citrus products; water and soda only make things worse!
Scoville Unit Ranking
- 100,000 or greater: Habanera, Scotch Bonnet, Jamaican Hot
- 50,000: Thai, Cayenne
- 10,000-20,000: Serrano
- 2,500-5,000: Jalapeno
- 1,000-1,500: Poblano
- 100-500: Pepperoncini (such as banana peppers)
- Bell, Italian

Pesto:
An Italian sauce originating in Genoa and made with fresh basil, pine nuts, Parmesan cheese, and oil. Delicious with carbohydrates such as pasta and bread.

Phyllo:
From the Greek for leaf, very thin pastry sheets used to make such dishes as baklava and spanakopita. Can be kept in the freezer for up to 1 year. Great for savory and sweet dishes alike.

Pomegranate:
A large fruit with a tough outer skin and edible seeds within. The seeds are the only edible part of this tart fruit. Pomegranates can be eaten fresh or as juice and are rich in Vitamin C and polyphenols. They are native in the regions from Iran to India. In the U.S., they are cultivated in California and Arizona.

Prosciutto:
Italian for ham, dried and cured, usually sliced thinly and served either raw or cooked. Salty and tender, it is usually served on an antipasto platter or wrapped around honeydew or cantaloupe as an appetizer.

Puff pastry:
A pastry made from butter, flour, and water. Found in the frozen section of the market or grocery store, it needs to be thawed before using. Beef Wellington and baked Brie both use puff pastry.

Puree:
To reduce to a smooth paste, often in a blender or food processor. Hummus, for example, is a dip made from pureeing chickpeas and other ingredients.

Puttanesca:
A hot, spicy Italian tomato sauce with capers, olives, anchovies, and a source of heat such as red pepper flakes or ground cayenne pepper. Usually served over spaghetti or other forms of pasta but would also be delicious over a hearty white fish like halibut or bass.

Quiche:
A pie, usually savory, that is made using butter crust, blind baked and then filled with custard of eggs, cream, and anything else you want. A classic quiche Lorraine is made with bacon.

Ratatouille:
A cooked eggplant, zucchini, onion, and tomato dish that can be served on the side or over a starch such as pasta or baked potatoes.

Roux:
A cooked mixture of equal parts flour and butter used as a thickening agent for making sauces like Béchamel or even a dish like classic New Orleans gumbo.

Saffron:
The most expensive spice in the world that is actually the dark orange stigmas of a type of crocus flower. Usually sold as threads and used to add incredible flavor to dishes. Only a small amount is needed at a time, so one bottle will get you a long way.

Salmonella:
Bacteria that can reside in meats, poultry, eggs, and other foods. Food must be cooked properly to a temperature of 165 degrees F to kill the bacteria and prevent illness.

Salt:
A mineral that is one of the most popular seasonings in the world.
   Forms Available:
· Sea salt: used as a finishing salt. Expensive, comes in a variety of textures and colors. Fleur de sel is a sea salt from France.

· Kosher salt: used today as traditional table salt was used in the past.
· Table salt: fine grain salt supplemented with iodine and anti-caking agents. Used less today by chefs due to the fact that it does not have a pure salt taste.

Sauté:
From the French verb sauter, "to jump," to sauté is to cook food quickly over high heat on the stovetop with a small amount of oil or butter. A sauté pan traditionally has a wide, flat bottom.

Savory:
A term used to describe a dish that does not contain sugar.

Sear:
To brown the surface of a food that is cooked by cooking on high heat. The process seals in juices and can be completed from rare to well done.

Serrated:
Description of a type of knife with 'teeth' that is ideal for cutting bread and tomatoes.

Shallot:
An onion that is milder, smaller, and sweeter than the traditional onion. Frequently used in French cooking.

Simple sugar:
A 50/50 mixture of sugar and water that is heated until the sugar dissolves. The mixture is then cooled and can be used to sweeten iced tea or coffee.

Simmer:
To cook food gently just below boiling after initially reaching the boiling point.

Spice:
Flavoring for food that comes from seeds, berries, bark, root, or fruit of a plant. Examples include: anise, cardamom, cumin, and ginger.

Steam:
To cook an item, usually vegetables, by placing it in metal or bamboo with a small amount of water..

Stone fruit:
Fruit whose seed is enclosed in a hard stone. Examples: mangos, peaches, plums, olives, cherries.

Sweat:
To cook vegetables over low heat in order to extract their moisture. Useful for vegetables that retain water.

Tapas:
Small appetizers, a term native to Spain.

Temper:
The process of mixing room temperature eggs or custard with hot liquid. The hot liquid is added to the egg mixture slowly to elevate the temperature of the mixture to prevent the eggs from scrambling. A vigorous whisking usually accompanies the process.

Thickening agents:
A combination of either water and cornstarch or water and flour added to thicken a soup or sauce.

Tofu:
A food product made from soybeans. Rich in protein, it does not contain lactose and is popular in vegetarian and vegan food as a substitute for meat and/or dairy.

Truffles:
A type of fungus, either white or black. The black truffles typically come from the Perigord region of France, from Italy, and from Saudi Arabia. In France pigs sniff them out, while in Saudi Arabia long walking sticks are used to locate them. Although they are expensive, only a small amount is needed to flavor a dish. Usually added to a finished dish either shaved or minced.

Truffle oil:
Olive oil infused with truffles; less expensive than using fresh truffles and can be drizzled.

Vanilla extract:
A liquid made by extracting vanilla flavor from vanilla beans using alcohol. It is not concentrated; only small amounts are needed. Typically used in baking but can flavor any dish.

Vinaigrette:
A dressing, usually for salads, which is classically made with oil, vinegar (or lemon juice as a replacement for the acid), mustard, salt, and pepper. The best way to make the dressing is either in a blender or with a whisk. First, combine the acid, mustard, salt, and pepper until well mixed. Then, add the oil in a slow drizzle. Oil to vinegar ratio is 3:1.

Whisk:
To mix a substance, usually eggs or cream, in a rapid whipping motion that incorporates air to produce meringue or whipped cream, for example.

Zest:
The outer rind of citrus fruit. Zesting refers to the process of obtaining the zest of a citrus fruit by using a cooking instrument called a microplane (often referred to as "zester"), which is essentially a very fine grater. Citrus zest is a wonderful garnish over fish, pasta, fruit, and desserts.

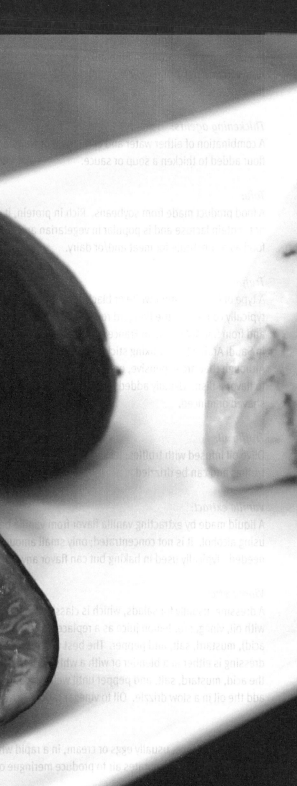

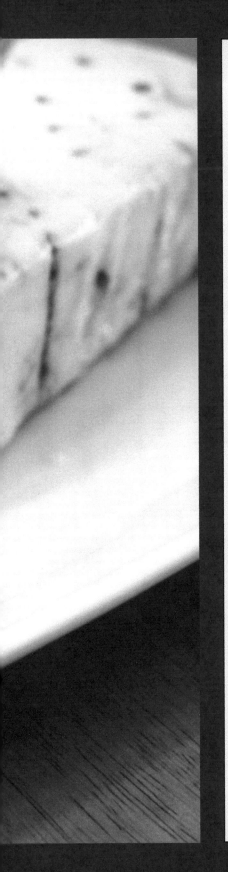

Classic Hummus

Roasted Veggie Dip

Sweet and Spicy Baked Brie

Spinach and Artichoke Dip

Honey Cashew Spread

New Orleans Oyster and Mushroom Paté, Two Ways

Quesadillas with Tropical Citrus Salsa

Toasted Cumin Pita Chips

Mediterranean Quiche

Basic Bruschetta

Fig and Gorgonzola Bites

Sweet Potato Crisps

Tapenade

Smoked Salmon Bites with Wasabi Cream Sauce

Baba Ganoush

Creamy Olive Dip

Mediterranean Sunset Spread

Tart á la Normandy

Classic Hummus

Are you a hummus lover? Sick of that store-bought taste?
Well now you can make your own hummus in less than fifteen minutes!
Perfect for a late night snack or as a starter for guests. You'll fool even
the most Mediterranean among them with our twist on this classic.

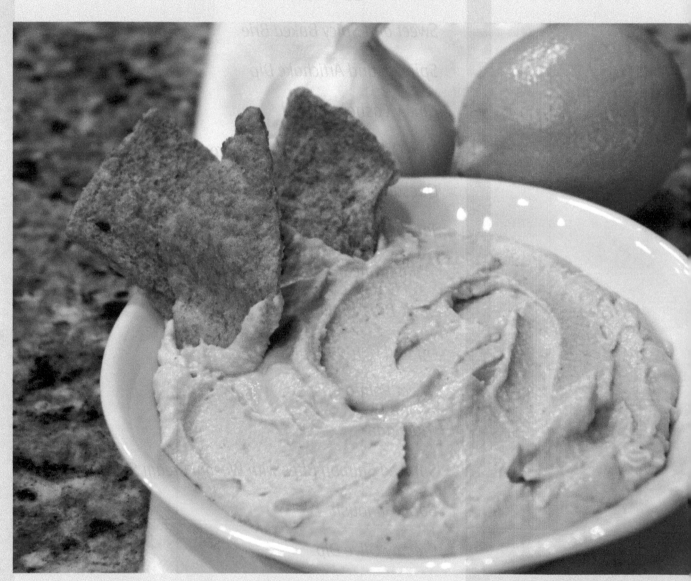

Servings: 6
Prep time: 10 minutes
Cooking time: 0
Cost: $2.12

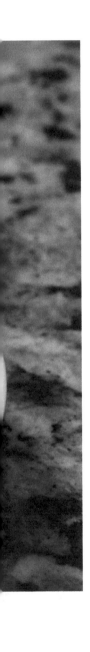

Ingredients

15 oz. can of garbanzo beans (chickpeas)
¼ cup bean juice (juice the chickpeas are packed in)
2 cloves garlic
¼ cup olive oil (+ extra for drizzling on top)
2 tablespoons of tahini (sesame seed paste)
Juice of 1 lemon (or ¼ cup lemon juice)
½ teaspoon of salt
½ teaspoon of ground black pepper
¼ teaspoon of cumin

Equipment

Food processor (2-cup or larger)
Strainer & bowl (for draining beans)
Measuring cups & spoons
Can opener

Directions

1. Drain the can of garbanzo beans (chickpeas) over a bowl to preserve the liquid.

2. You'll be using ¼ cup later in the blending process, so don't throw it away!

3. Put the garlic in the food processor and pulse for 10 seconds. Add the garbanzo beans, bean juice, and olive oil and blend until it starts to become smooth. Add the tahini and the juice of 1 lemon (about ¼ cup). You can use either fresh or jarred lemon juice.

4. Add salt, pepper, and cumin, and let the machine run for 2 minutes. We like to drizzle the finished hummus with olive oil to add extra flavor. Serve with our toasted cumin pita chips.

ROASTED VEGGIE DIP

This dish is a delicious hors d'oeuvre any time of the year. It's a great choice for potluck parties—easy to make and transport, and can be made ahead of time. It's rich and light at the same time! This recipe uses one of our favorite reusable ingredients: tomato paste in a tube. It comes in a 4.5 oz. tube with a cap and can be stored in the fridge for easy reuse. You can find it in the Italian/pasta aisle of the supermarket.

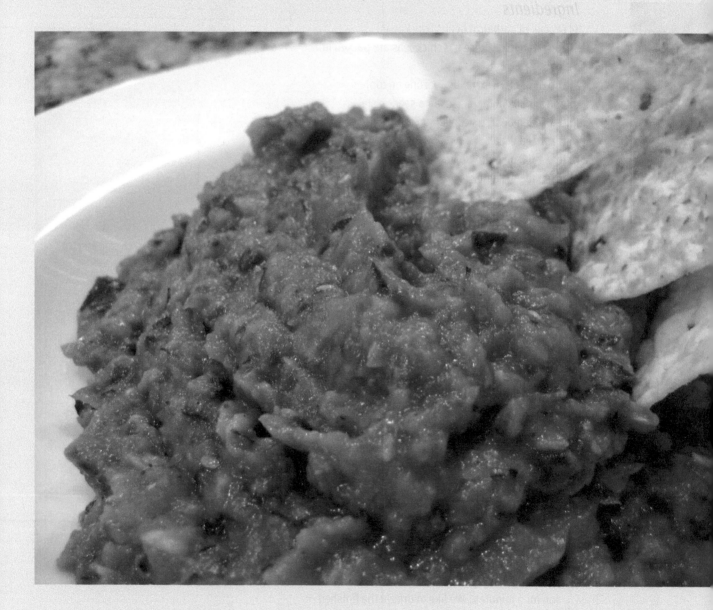

Servings: 8 – 10
Prep time: 15 minutes
Cooking time: 45 minutes
Cost: $8.22

Ingredients

1 red bell pepper
1 yellow bell pepper
1 eggplant
1 red onion
1 zucchini
¼ cup + 2 tablespoons olive oil
2 tablespoons balsamic vinegar
2 tablespoons honey
2 tablespoons tomato paste (tube or can)
2 teaspoons salt
1 teaspoon black pepper
1 bag corn chips

Equipment

2-cup food processor (or larger if you have it)
Cutting board & knife
Roasting pan
Large mixing bowl
Measuring cups & spoons

Directions

1. Preheat the oven to 375 degrees F.

2. After rinsing and trimming all the vegetables,
   give them a rough chop.
   No peeling is necessary for this dish!
   Distribute the veggies evenly on a roasting pan.
   If you want to eliminate a minor stage of cleanup,
   place a sheet of parchment paper on the roasting
   pan before adding the vegetables.
   Once they are laid out, drizzle ¼ cup of olive oil
   over them. Then sprinkle them with 1 teaspoon
   of salt and ½ teaspoon of pepper.
   Proceed to mix them—we recommend using your
   hands. They really are your best kitchen tools!

3. After the oven has preheated, slip the pan in and
   bake for 40 minutes, until they are "fork tender"
   (a fork will slide easily in and out of the food).

4. The next stage involves the food processor.
   Don't forget that for food to blend properly, it requires
   some kind of liquid. We recommend blending the
   vegetables in four batches if you have a 2-cup food
   processor.
   You can do it in fewer with a larger food processor.
   Blend each stage for about 30 seconds.
   Add 2 tablespoons of honey to the first batch and
   blend until smooth. Empty the pureed contents
   into a large mixing or serving bowl.
   Add 2 tablespoons of tomato paste to the second
   batch and blend for another 30 seconds.
   Remove the dip and place in the bowl.
   Repeat this process for the last two batches, this time
   adding 2 tablespoons of balsamic vinegar to the
   third batch and 2 tablespoons of olive oil to the fourth
   batch for 30 seconds each.
   Each batch will be a different color once pureed—
   don't worry, when you mix all batches at the end the
   color will be beautiful.

5. Serve with corn chips or pita chips and enjoy!

SWEET & SPICY BAKED BRIE

What we love most about this dish, besides how simple it is to make, is its versatility! Follow our suggestions for a delicious and easy appetizer that will stimulate the taste buds of all your buddies and will surely show your parents that you learned something for all the money they put into your education! This affordable basic hors d'oeuvre can be modified to include any garnish or spread you think would go well with Brie! For instance, if you're up for sautéing some mushrooms, you'll have a hearty opening for an autumn feast. Whatever you can imagine, you can do after you follow our basic steps.

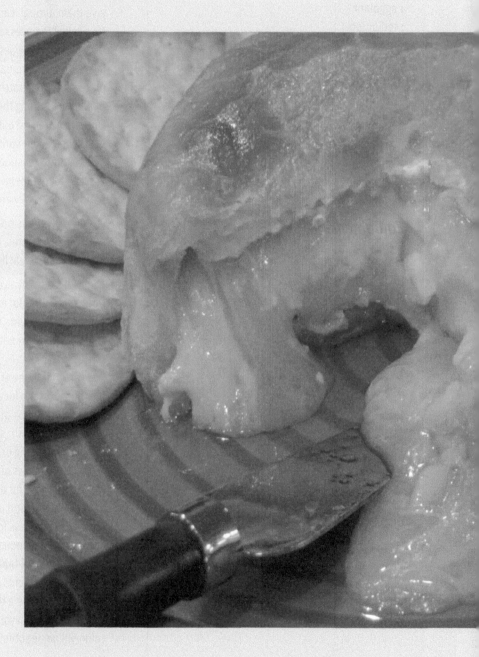

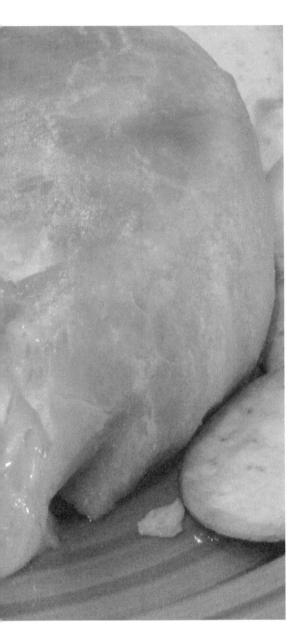

Servings: 6 - 8
Cooking time: 15 minutes
Prep time: 15 minutes
Cost: $18.44

Ingredients

1 sheet of puff pastry (comes frozen)
1 8 oz. round of Brie
1 jar of red pepper jelly
1 egg, beaten
All-purpose flour, about 2 tablespoons (for rolling out pastry)
Water crackers

Equipment

Baking sheet
Rolling pin
Pastry brush (if you don't have one, a spoon will work)
Whisk (if you don't have one, a fork will work)
Parchment paper

Directions

1. Thaw the puff pastry as per directions on the package. Preheat the oven to 400 degrees F.

2. First, you want to dust your working surface, hands, and rolling pin generously with flour to make sure the puff pastry does not stick.
   Use your rolling pin to roll it out into a large, thin piece that will accommodate the size of your Brie. Be sure not to leave the pastry too thick, or else the Brie will not soften. Place the round of Brie on the center of the square and fold each corner over the brie. There will be about 1/3 excess dough—cut it off and save it as a garnish or decoration for the top of the brie (you can shape the dough however you want or even use a cookie cutter for special designs). Place the brie seam-side down on a baking sheet covered with parchment. Baked brie makes for a messy cleanup, so using parchment paper is extremely helpful in this recipe.

3. Beat one fresh egg in a small bowl. Add 2 tablespoons of water and whisk again (this is now called an egg wash! Take the pastry brush and glaze the top and sides of the brie with the egg wash. If you don't have a pastry brush, just spoon the egg onto the brie and use the back side of the spoon to spread the egg wash gently over the dough. Place the baking sheet in the preheated oven.

4. Bake for 15 minutes, until the crust is golden brown. The Brie is ready to serve with red pepper jelly and crackers or however else you might envision it.

SPINACH & ARTICHOKE DIP

Your friends will devour this rich, tasty dip. Everyone loves to order this dip at restaurants, now you can make it at home. This is what we call comfort food with some healthy additions for guilt free enjoyment. Serve with tortilla chips, pita chips, or crusty bread.

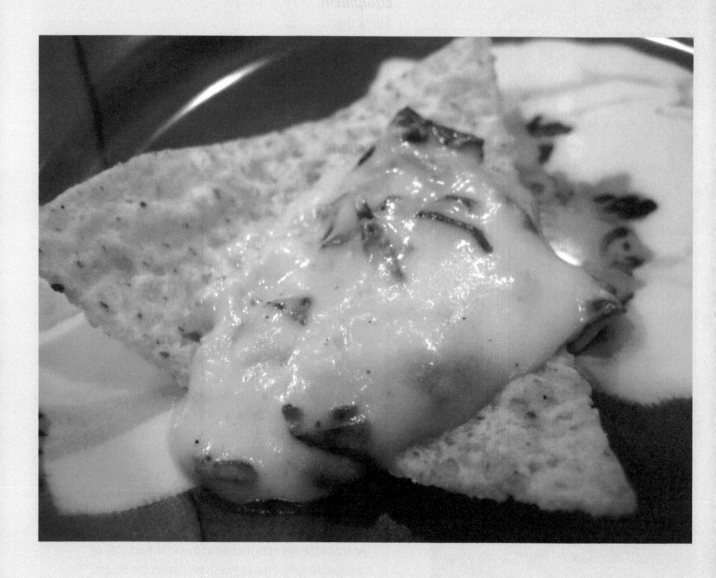

Servings: 8 – 10
Prep time: 10 minutes
Cook time: 15 minutes
Cost: $12.73

Ingredients
4 tablespoons unsalted butter
4 tablespoons all-purpose flour
2 cups milk *
6 ounce bag fresh spinach leaves (triple washed)
14 oz can artichoke hearts
1 tablespoon garlic paste
1 teaspoon salt
1 teaspoon pepper
½ cup Parmesan
2 cups shredded mozzarella (comes in plastic packages)

Equipment
Cutting board & knife
Saucepan
Stirring spoon
Measuring cups & spoons

Directions
1. Chop the spinach and artichoke on a cutting board.

2. Melt the butter in a saucepan over medium-low heat. Once the
    butter has melted add the flour and whisk for 2-3 minutes until
    combined and is blonde in color (you have made a blonde roux,
    which is a commonly used base for thickening sauces).
    Slowly add the milk (adding in small increments helps the mixture to
    gain a smooth consistency). Bring the sauce to a boil over medium-
    high heat. Once it boils, turn the heat down to medium-low. Add
    the spinach, artichokes, cheese, garlic, salt, and pepper and cook
    for 8-10 minutes until thick. Serve warm.

3. Many cooking experts advocate using milk that is warmed but you
    can make this sauce with cold milk as well—we've tried it both
    ways. There is a risk of having lumps in your sauce if you use
    cold milk.

HONEY CASHEW SPREAD

You will want to serve this at every party you have. Whenever we put this one on the table, our friends and family go crazy over this nutty, crunchy, smoky spread. Serve it with our toasted cumin pita chips for a smoky explosion.

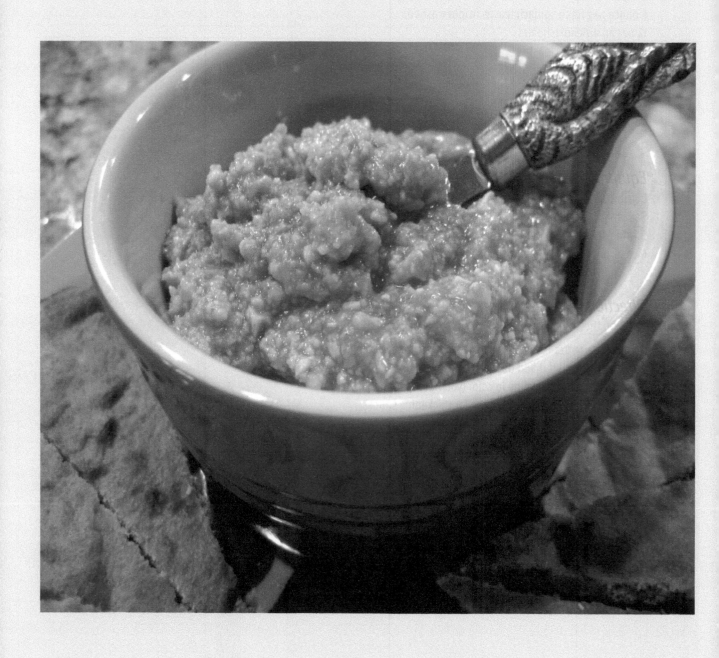

Servings: 6 – 8
Prep time: 5 minutes
Cook time: 0 minutes
Cost: $5.71

Ingredients

1 cup of cashew nuts (if salted, do not add any extra
salt; if not then add ½ teaspoon Kosher salt)
¼ cup olive oil
2 tablespoons honey
1 teaspoon cumin
2 teaspoons garlic paste
½ teaspoon ground black pepper

Equipment

Food processor
Measuring cups & spoons

Directions

Mix all ingredients in a food processor for 10 to 20
seconds, then add the olive oil in a slow stream to the
food processor while it is running. Let the processor run
for about 1 minute.

*Tip: if you have nonstick cooking spray around, spray
the measuring spoon before you add the honey, and the
honey will slide off the spoon

NEW ORLEANS OYSTER AND MUSHROOM PATÉ, TWO WAYS

Oyster paté two ways! Whether you're using leftover raw oysters or oysters from a can, we've concocted some tasty, simple recipes to make your get-together that much more elegant.

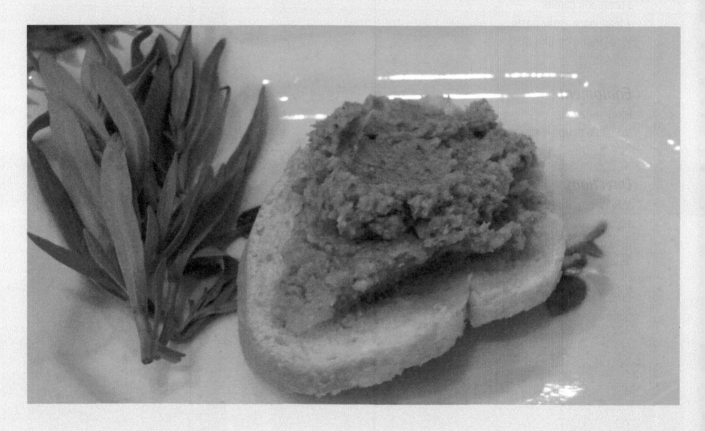

With Fresh Oysters
Servings: 4 – 6
Prep time: 5 minutes
Cooking time: 15 minutes
Cost: $14.77

With Fresh Oysters

Ingredients

8 oz. shucked raw oysters, chopped
    (about 8 medium oysters)
1 cup white button mushrooms, chopped
¼ yellow onion, chopped
1 tablespoon garlic paste
1 tablespoon chopped tarragon
¼ cup oyster juice (reserved from oysters)
2 tablespoons olive oil
2 tablespoons unsalted butter, chilled
¼ cup bread crumbs

Equipment

Sauté pan
Food processor
Measuring cups & spoons

Directions

1. Chop the oysters, removing the tough stem, and reserve ¼ of the oyster juice.

2. Heat a sauté pan over medium heat with 2 tablespoons of olive oil. Pour in the chopped quarter of an onion and allow it to sweat for about 3 minutes. Add the mushrooms and garlic paste and cook for another 5 minutes. Add the oysters and reserved ¼ cup of the oyster juice and sauté over medium-low heat for 10 minutes.

3. Remove the pan from the stove and let the oysters cool for 5 minutes. Then add oyster-mushroom mixture to the food processor. Blend for about 15 seconds, then add the tarragon and breadcrumbs and blend again for 10 seconds. Add the butter, one tablespoon at a time, blending in turns. Blend for 30 seconds, scoop into a small bowl, and allow to set in the fridge for several hours.

4. Serve with crusty bread or water crackers.

With Smoked Oysters
Servings: 4 – 6
Prep time: 5 minutes
Cooking time: 8 minutes
Cost: $4.62

With Smoked Oysters

Ingredients

1 x 3 oz. can smoked oysters (packed in oil)
1 cup sliced prewashed mushrooms
1 scallion (green onion), chopped, green part only
1 teaspoon olive oil
1 teaspoon garlic paste
½ cup plain cream cheese
1/8 teaspoon black pepper

Equipment

Food processor
Small sauté pan
Measuring cups & spoons

Directions

1. Sauté the mushrooms with olive oil, pepper, garlic paste, and chopped green onion (green part only) over medium-low heat for 8 minutes. Set aside.

2. Drain the can of smoked oysters (they're saturated in oil!). Put the oysters and sautéed mushrooms into the food processor and blend for 15 seconds. Add the cream cheese and blend again for about 30 seconds. Scoop out, set in a dish in the fridge for several hours, then serve either with plain, toasted baguette slices or plain water crackers.

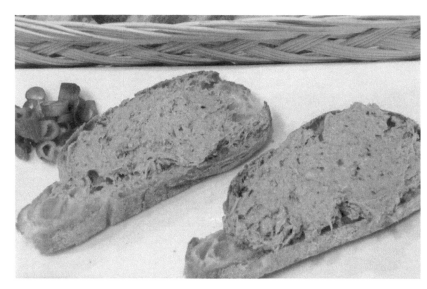

QUESADILLAS WITH TROPICAL CITRUS SALSA

Give this Mexican staple a tropical zing with our special citrus salsa.
This fusion of zesty cheese and tangy fruit flavors is light enough to start
a party with, but it comes with warning: get one before they're gone!

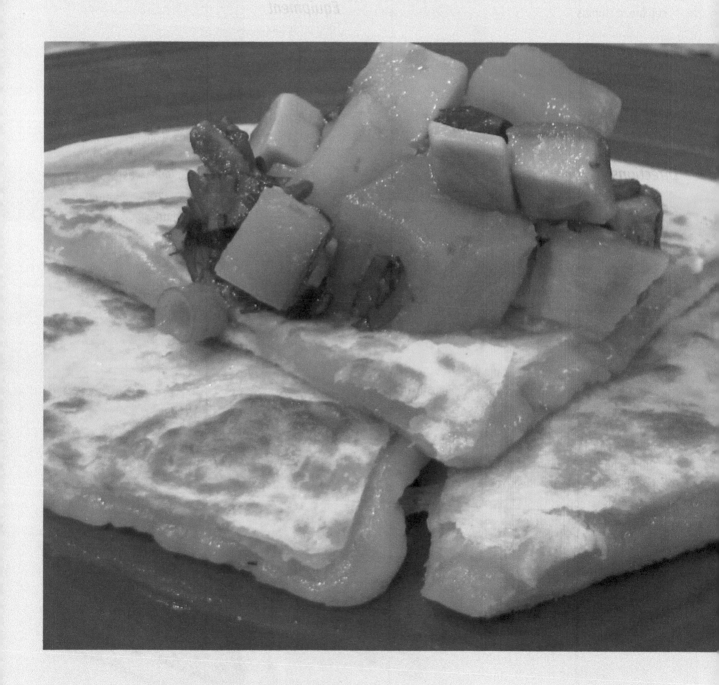

Servings: 8 – 10
Prep time: 15 minutes
Cooking time: 4 minutes
Cost: $14.84

Ingredients

1 yellow pepper diced
1 ripe papaya (small) diced
1 avocado diced
2 green onions chopped (green parts only)
1 mango diced
1 package 10 soft taco tortilla shells (8 inch size)
1 x 8 oz pack shredded mozzarella
1 x 8 oz pack shredded sharp cheddar
2 tablespoons lime juice
2 tablespoons lemon juice
2 tablespoons chopped cilantro
1 teaspoon salt
5 squirts hot sauce
5 teaspoons oil (for cooking the quesadillas)

Equipment

1 medium-size mixing bowl
Cutting board
Chopping knife
Sauté or fry pan
Measuring spoons

Directions

For the citrus salsa:

1. Peel and scoop out the black seeds of the papaya.
   Dice the yellow pepper, papaya, avocado, and mango.

2. Chop the green parts of the green onions into small pieces and 2 tablespoons of cilantro.

3. Secret tip: A helpful way to preserve counter space is by adding ingredients to the mixing bowl as you've chopped or diced them. Mea sure out 2 tablespoons of lemon juice, ¼ cup of lime juice, and pour both into the bowl with the fruit. Add the hot sauce. Mix together with a spoon. Sprinkle with 1 teaspoon of salt. Mix and set aside.

For the quesadillas:

1. Heat the pan over medium heat. Take a tortilla and sprinkle with ½ cup of mozzarella and ½ cup cheddar and cover with another tortilla. (You can really use any combination of cheese you like in this dish.)

2. Add 1teaspoon oil to the hot pan and place the quesadilla in the pan and cook for 1 minute per side. Cut into quarters or eighths and serve with salsa.

TOASTED CUMIN PITA CHIPS

Their crunchy, firm texture makes these chips ideal for any one of our many homemade spreads. Replace those pricey store-bought pita chips with our fresh ones! Yia-Yia, our resident Mediterranean grandmother, says they are incomparable!

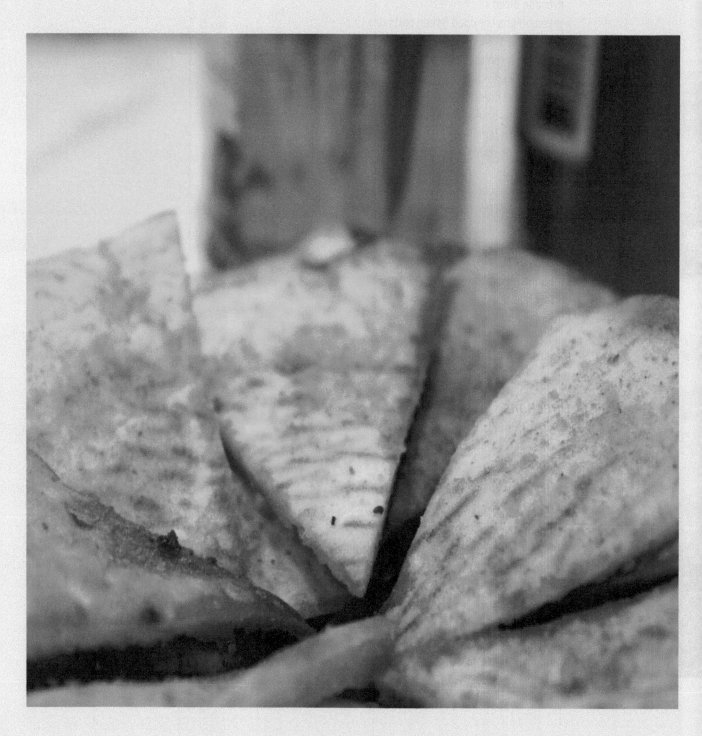

Servings: 6 – 8
Prep time: 10 minutes
Cooking time: 4 – 5 minutes
Cost: $2.46

Ingredients

4 pitas
¼ cup olive oil
1 teaspoon garlic paste
1 teaspoon cumin

Equipment

Mixing bowl
Baking sheet
Pastry brush
Whisk (or fork)
Parchment paper (optional)

Directions

1. Preheat the oven to 400 degrees F.

2. Cut pita bread rounds in eighths and place on a baking sheet. Time saving tip: Layer several pitas before slicing in order to cut more pieces at one time. Mix together the olive oil, garlic paste, and cumin with a whisk.

3. Brush the pita with the olive oil mixture and bake for 5 - 6 minutes until golden and crusty.

4. Sprinkle the freshly baked pitas with salt and serve immediately, either alone or with a dip of your choice!

MEDITERRANEAN QUICHE

These small tarts are a great snack or as a starter for a Mediterranean meal. You'll love the combination of the nuttiness of the chickpeas and the sweetness of the spinach. This is basically a mini quiche.
You can substitute the vegetables and beans for crab and tarragon or broccoli and cheddar.

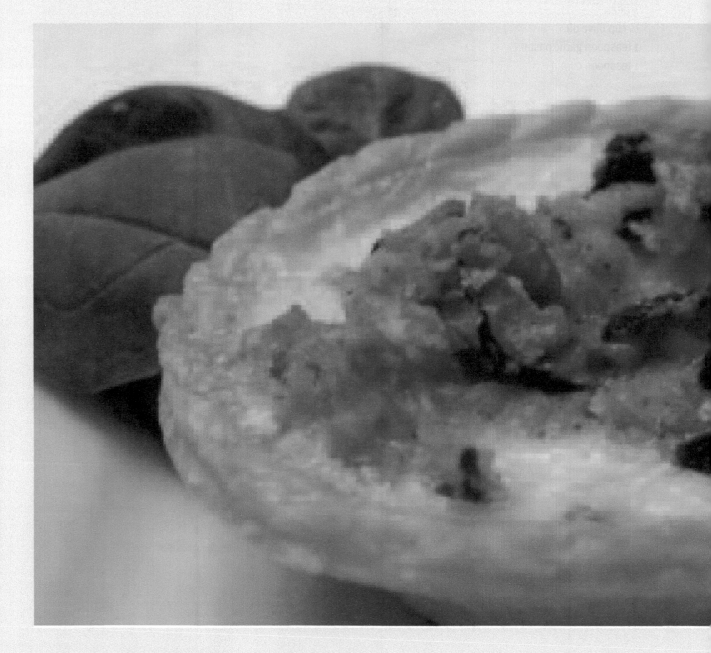

Servings: 8
Prep time: 10 minutes
Cooking time: 30 minutes
Cost: $ 9.74

Ingredients
1 package of 8 pastry shells (in the frozen food section)
1 zucchini, diced
½ medium onion, chopped
14 oz. can chickpeas (garbanzo beans)
1 teaspoon garlic paste
1 teaspoon lemon juice
2 teaspoons salt (divided)
1 teaspoon black pepper (divided)
2 cups spinach
1 tablespoon cumin
2 eggs
½ cup heavy cream

Equipment
Medium size sauté pan
Mixing bowls
Measuring cups & spoons

Directions
1. Preheat the oven to 375 degrees F.

2. Thaw pastry shells according to the package directions.

3. Sauté spinach, zucchini, onion, garlic paste, cumin, 1 teaspoon salt, and ½ teaspoon pepper over medium heat for about 8 to 10 minutes. In a separate bowl, mash the chickpeas and add lemon juice. Add the cooked spinach mixture and mix thoroughly.

4. In a mixing bowl, combine the eggs, cream, 1 teaspoon salt, and ½ teaspoon pepper.

5. Place a heaping tablespoon of the spinach-chickpea mixture in the bottom of each pastry shell and fill shells with egg-cream mixture. Bake for 20 minutes.

6. Serve warm or at room temperature. (It's also delicious cold for breakfast!)

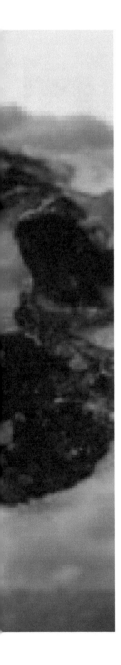

BASIC BRUSCHETTA (BRU-SKE-TA)

Who says you need to go to an Italian restaurant to have authentic Italian bruschetta? Believe us, our bruschetta recipe will make you feel like you're sitting in a sidewalk café in Siena—without the hassle of leaving your own kitchen! Using simple ingredients, we've created a refreshing, crunchy appetizer for a lazy afternoon or an evening with friends.

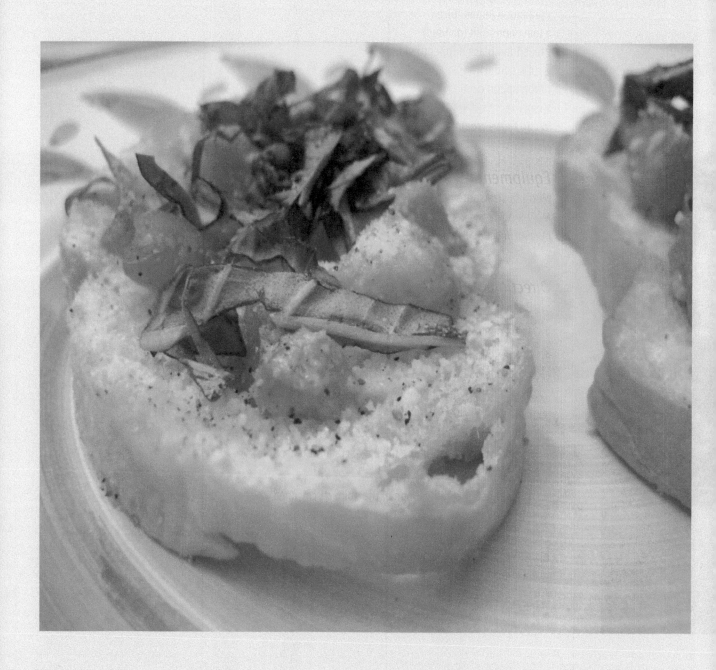

Servings: 4
Prep time: 15 minutes
Cooking time: 8 minutes
Cost: $ 5.62

Ingredients
½ loaf Italian bread (8 slices for 4 people)
2 tomatoes, diced
1 clove garlic
2 tablespoons olive oil + extra for brushing
1 teaspoon salt
½ teaspoon black pepper
½ teaspoon Parmesan per slice
4 fresh basil leaves

Equipment
Cutting board
Serrated knife
Paring knife
Baking sheet
Mixing bowl
Measuring cups & spoons

Directions
1. Preheat oven to 400 degrees F.

2. Dice 1 large ripe tomato on a cutting board.
   Pour into a mixing bowl with the olive oil, salt,
   and pepper.

3. Slice the bread into ½ inch thick slices.
   Arrange over parchment paper on a baking sheet.
   Drizzle with olive oil and put in the oven for 1
   minute only. Remove immediately.
   Brush with a freshly cut clove of garlic, top with
   the tomatoes, sprinkle each slice with ½ teaspoon
   Parmesan, and put back in the oven for 7 minutes.

4. On a cutting board, chiffonade 3 or 4 fresh basil
   leaves. Place over the bruschetta slices once
   they are out of the oven, sprinkle with salt
   and pepper if desired, and serve hot!

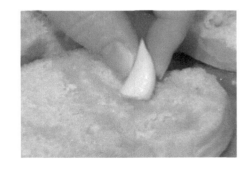

Fig and Gorgonzola Bites

Want to impress your friends? Significant other? Professor? This ridiculously low maintenance appetizer instantly adds gourmet flair to any meal. It's a great late night bite also—the taste combination of the salty Gorgonzola cheese and sweet fig spread is amazing! You'll have a fantastic nibbler in a matter of mere minutes.

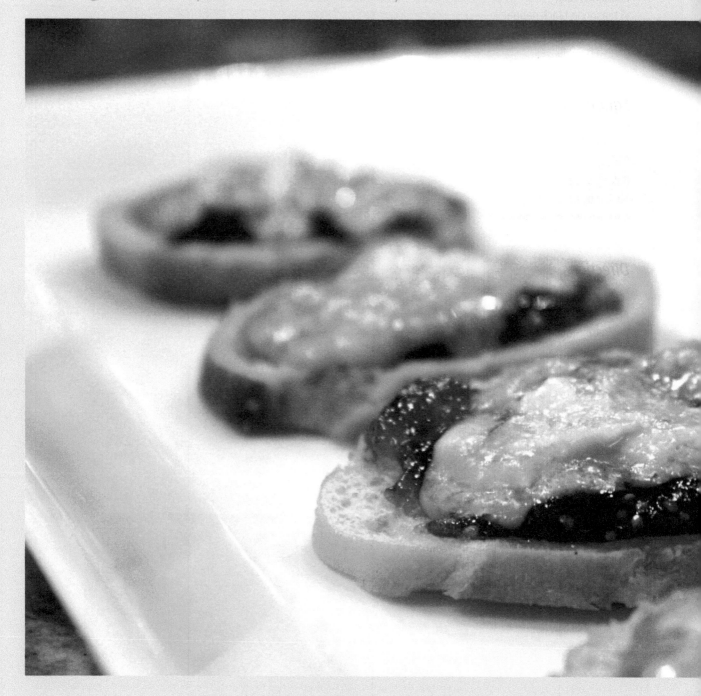

Servings: 6-8
Prep time: 5 minutes
Cook time: 4 minutes
Cost: $ 11.92

Ingredients
1 fresh baguette (makes about 40-50 ¼ inch slices,
depending on the length of your baguette)
Fig spread (comes in 8.5 oz. jars)
8 ounces Gorgonzola cheese, softened
2 tablespoons unsalted butter, softened

Equipment
Baking sheet
Large slicing knife
Small mixing bowl
Parchment paper (optional)

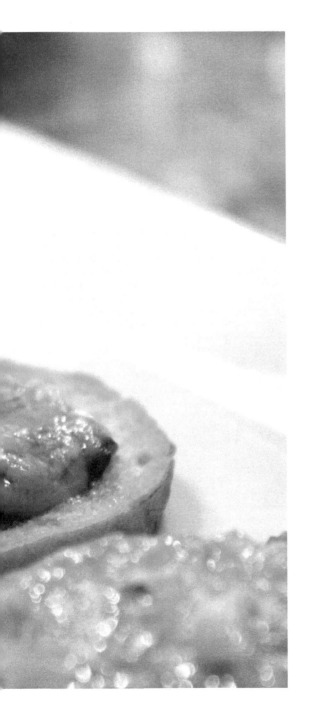

Directions
1. Before you do anything else, let the Gorgonzola and butter
   sit out for at least an hour prior to your baking time.

2. Preheat the oven to 400 degrees F.

3. In a bowl, mix the Gorgonzola and butter and set aside.

4. When you are ready to begin, cut the baguette into ¼ inch
   thick slices. Arrange them on the baking sheet.
   Put the baguette slices in the oven for 2 minutes.
   As soon as the time has passed, take them out, but leave
   the oven on; you will be using it again shortly!

5. Drop ½ teaspoon of the fig spread onto each baguette slice
   and spread accordingly.
   Then place a ½ teaspoon of the Gorgonzola and butter mix
   on top of the fig spread. Depending on how strongly you
   want your bites to taste of Gorgonzola, you can apply more
   or less to each bite. Just keep in mind that the slices are about
   to go back into the oven, so try not to overload them!

6. Place the baguette slices into the oven again for 2 minutes.
   Remove, arrange on a plate, e voila! A gourmet touch to any meal.

7. If Gorgonzola's flavor is too strong for you, you can substitute
   blue cheese. It is equally delicious, just a little milder.

SWEET POTATO CRISPS

Not your average potato chip. Thinly sliced sweet potatoes get smothered in delicious layers of flavoring and baked in the oven for a homemade, healthy treat. Wonderful as a side dish to a meal, great as a finger food for guests, and perfect for a midnight snack. Never open a bag of potato chips again!

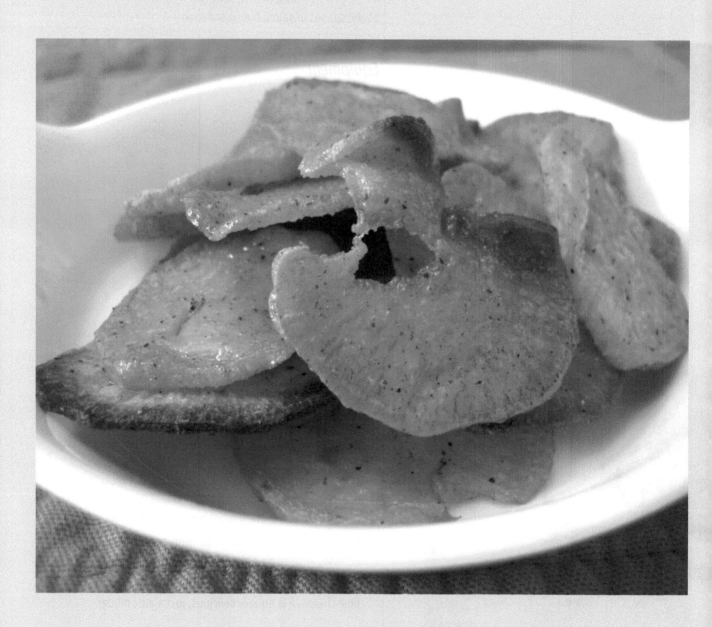

Servings: 6 - 8
Prep time: 10 minutes
Cook time: 20 minutes
Cost: $2.50

Ingredients

1 large sweet potato
1/3 cup olive oil
¼ teaspoon salt (divided)
½ teaspoon pepper
¼ teaspoon cinnamon

Equipment

Baking sheet
Mixing bowl
Measuring cups & spoons

Directions

1. Preheat the oven to 400 degrees F.

2. Wash and peel sweet potato. Cut the potato into thin slices. Be sure to make the slices as thin as possible for ultimate crispness.

3. Place the sweet potato slices in a large bowl and add olive oil, ½ teaspoon each of salt, pepper, and cinnamon and mix until slices are evenly coated.

4. Place on a baking sheet and bake until crispy, about 20 minutes.

TAPENADE

No one can refuse this spread. Tried and tested on many different friends and family members, we guarantee this dish will be the talk of the town for a week.

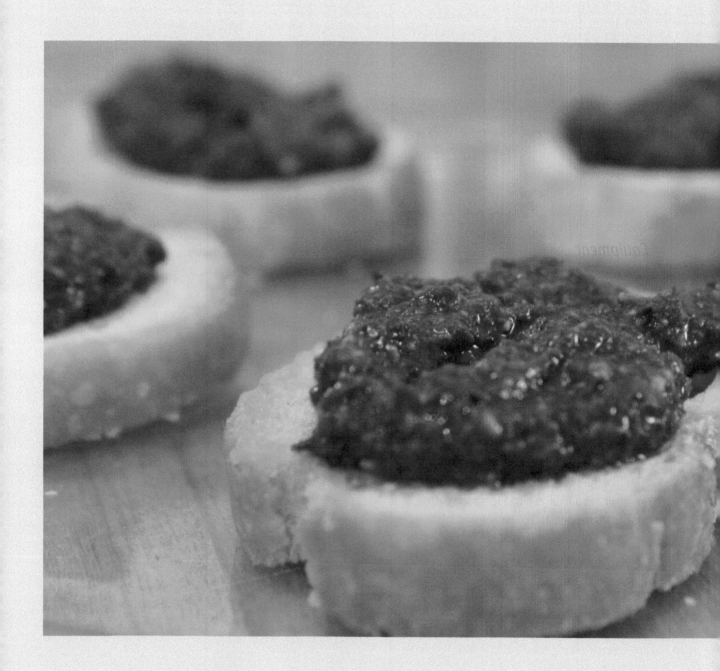

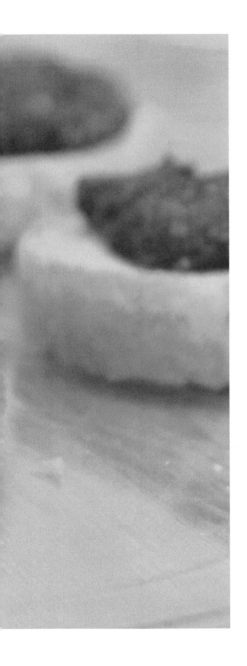

Servings: 4 – 6
Prep time: 2 minutes
Cooking time: 1 minute
Cost: $7.22

Ingredients
1 cup Kalamata olives, pitted
3 tablespoons capers
¼ cup olive oil
1 teaspoon Dijon mustard
2 tablespoons pine nuts
¼ teaspoon black pepper

Equipment
Food processor
Baking sheet
Measuring spoons

Directions
1. Preheat the oven to broil.

2. Combine all the ingredients in a food processor and blend for 30 seconds, less for chunkier spread.

3. Thinly slice a baguette and drizzle with olive oil, then put under a preheated broiler for just about 1 minute. Once the bread begins to brown, remove the bread, spread with tapenade, and serve.

SMOKED SALMON BITES WITH WASABI CREAM SAUCE

You'll love these fast, easy, and delicious hors d'oeuvres. They are wonderful for parties. A sure fire crowd pleaser.

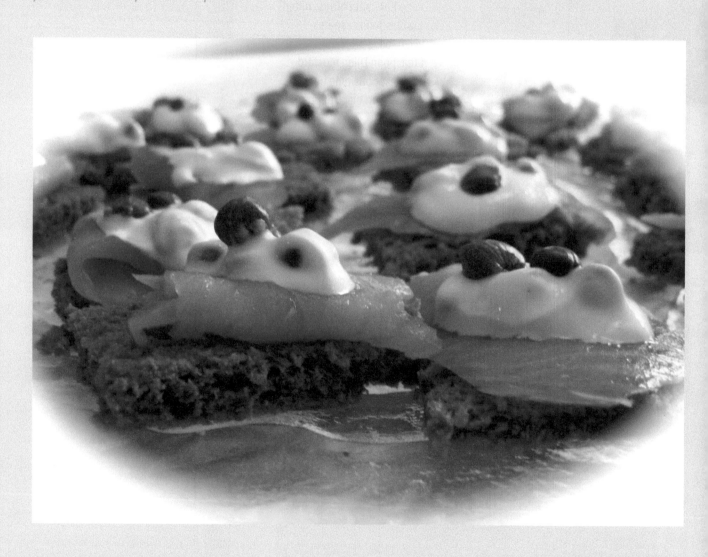

Servings: 4 - 6
Prep time: 10 minutes
Cook time: none
Cost: $8.00

Ingredients

4 oz. package of smoked salmon
¼ cup capers, drained
3 heaping tablespoons sour cream
1 tablespoon lemon juice
1 teaspoon wasabi paste or horseradish
5 slices of pumpernickel or rye bread

Equipment

Serrated knife
Mixing bowl

Directions

Cut the crusts off the bread and slice each piece into
quarters. You will have 20 quarters. Place a small piece
of smoked salmon on each quarter. In a mixing bowl,
mix together the sour cream wasabi paste and lemon juice.
Add the capers and mix gently. Place a dollop of the wasabi
caper cream sauce on each piece of salmon and serve.
You can garnish with fresh dill if you have it in your fridge
or herb garden.

BABA GANOUSH

We've added a bit of sweetness to this traditional Middle Eastern dish. It's incredibly easy to make and great if you have leftover eggplants from another recipe, like the Athens or Istanbul dinner.

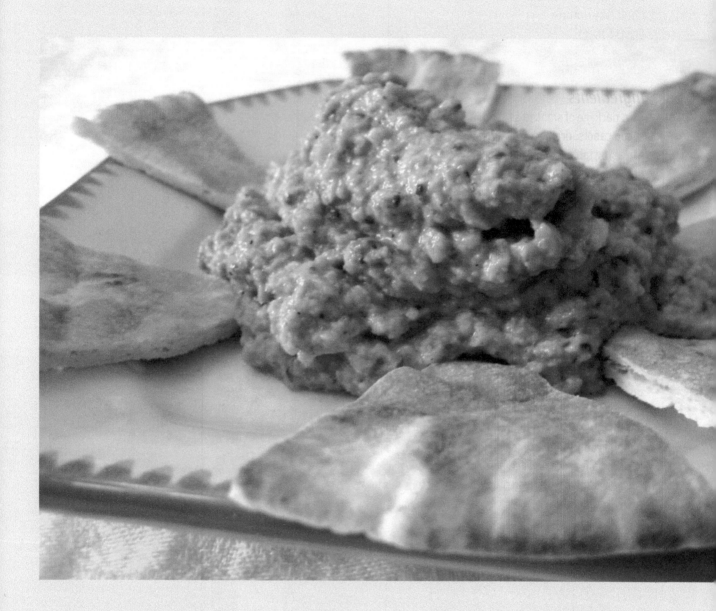

Servings: 6 – 8
Prep time: 10 minutes
Cooking time: 45 minutes
Cost: $3.37

Ingredients

1 large eggplant
3 teaspoons tahini paste (mix thoroughly before
scooping it out)
1 teaspoon garlic paste
¼ teaspoon cumin
½ teaspoon salt
¼ teaspoon pepper
¼ teaspoon paprika
1 tablespoon olive oil
1 tablespoon fig spread
¼ cup lemon juice

Equipment

Food processor
Baking sheet
Cutting Board
Chopping knife
Measuring cups & spoons

Directions

1. Preheat the oven to 375 degrees F.

2. About 1 hour before serving the baba
   ganoush, cut three slits along the
   eggplant and place in the preheated
   oven for 45 minutes. Once it's done, remove
   and allow it to cool for another 15 minutes.

3. Remove the skin and chop the meat of the
   eggplant into small chunks. Place in the
   food processor along with the other
   ingredients and blend until smooth, about
   30 seconds. Serve warm or cooled with
   pita bread.

CREAMY OLIVE DIP

This light, summery dip is so refreshing. It has all the flavors of the Mediterranean—olives, feta, figs, and artichokes. Dip potato chips, pita wedges, or veggies. Spread the leftovers on a roast beef sandwich. Mmm!

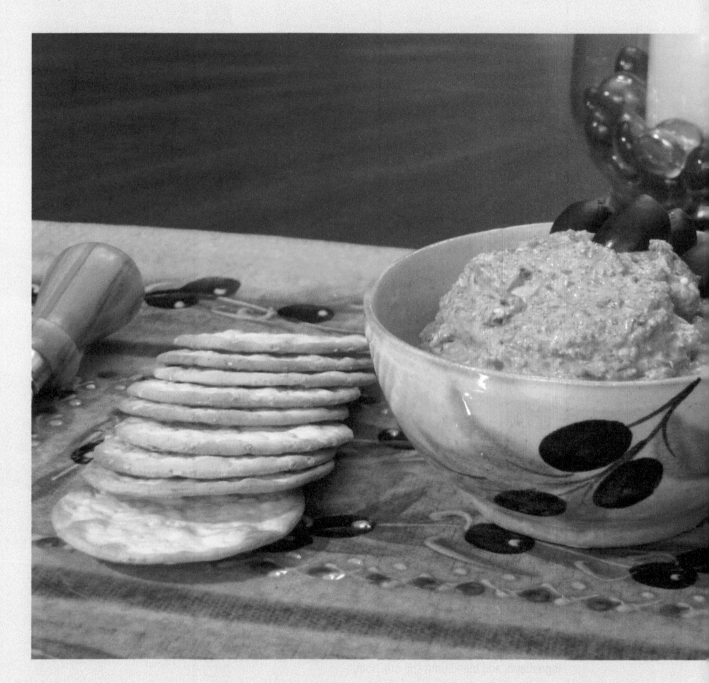

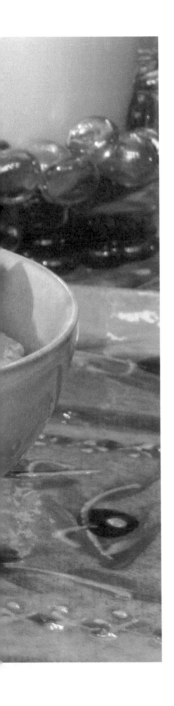

Servings: 6 - 8
Prep time: 1 minute
Cooking time: 0 minutes
Cost: $ 10.63

Ingredients
1 cup Kalamata olives
1 cup feta cheese
½ cup sour cream
1 tablespoon fig spread
3 artichoke hearts
½ teaspoon ground black pepper

Equipment
Food processor
Measuring cups & spoons

Directions
Combine ingredients in food processor and blend until smooth.

MEDITERRANEAN SUNSET SPREAD

This spread is so refreshing! It's great on a summer day. You can serve it with a baguette or with pita chips or fresh veggies. You can substitute cream cheese for the sour cream for a milder, less tangy taste.

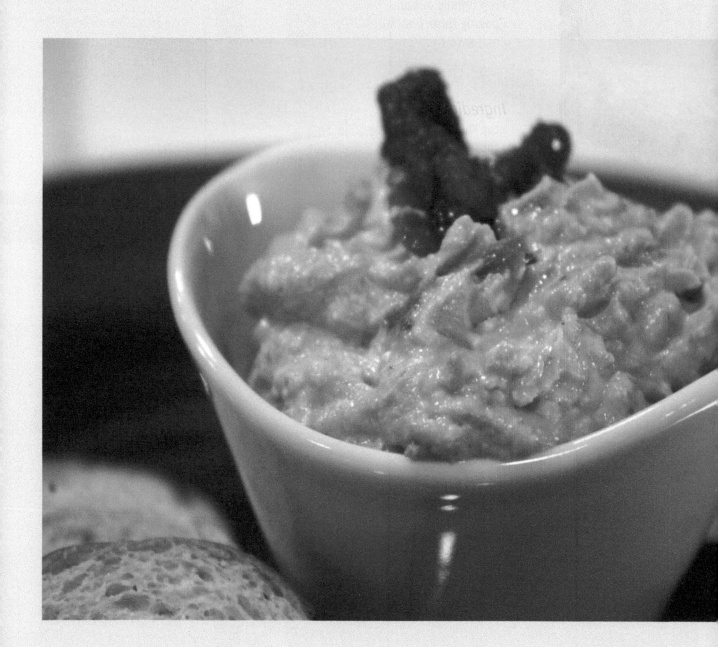

Servings: 6 - 8
Prep time: 5 minutes
Cook time: 0 minutes
Cost: $10.25

Ingredients
1 cup feta cheese
½ cup sundried tomatoes, drained (comes in jars packed in oil)
½ cup sour cream
2 tablespoons olive oil
1 tablespoon lemon juice
¼ teaspoon black pepper
1 baguette, sliced

Equipment
2-cup food processor

Directions
Place all ingredients in a food processor and blend until smooth. Spread over slices of baguette. You can also serve this spread with our homemade pita chips.

TART À LA NORMANDY

Consider this your first class ticket to France.

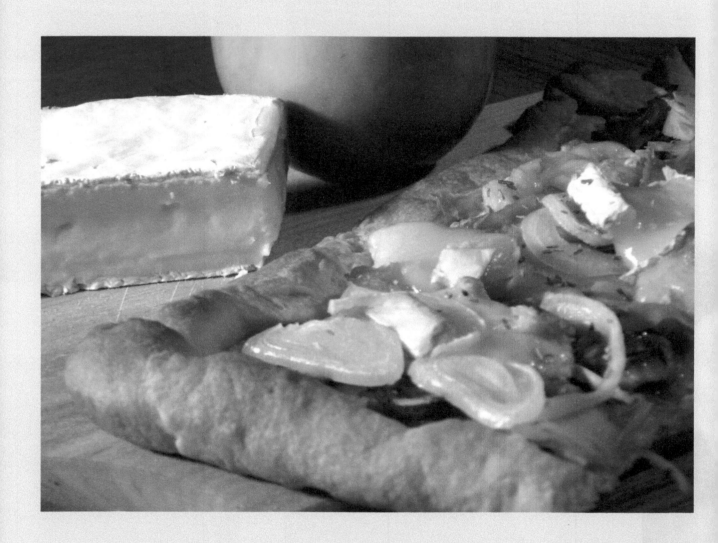

Servings: 4 - 6
Prep time: 10 minutes
Cooking time: 15 minutes
Cost: $ 9.50

Ingredients
1 can of thin crust pizza dough
½ granny smith apple, thinly sliced
1 cup baby portabella mushrooms, sliced thinly
1 shallot, thinly sliced
4 oz. brie, cubed into small pieces
3 slices of ham, chiffonade
½ tsp rosemary

Equipment
Baking sheet
Measuring cups & spoons

Directions
1. Preheat the oven according to package directions. After you have pre-baked the crust and prepared the ingredients, lightly drizzle olive oil over the dough and distribute evenly with the back of a spoon.

2. Place the prepared ingredients on the dough in the following order:
   Mushrooms
   Apples
   Ham
   Brie
   Shallots

3. Sprinkle rosemary on top. Return to the oven and bake until the edges are golden brown, about 10 – 15 minutes depending on package directions.

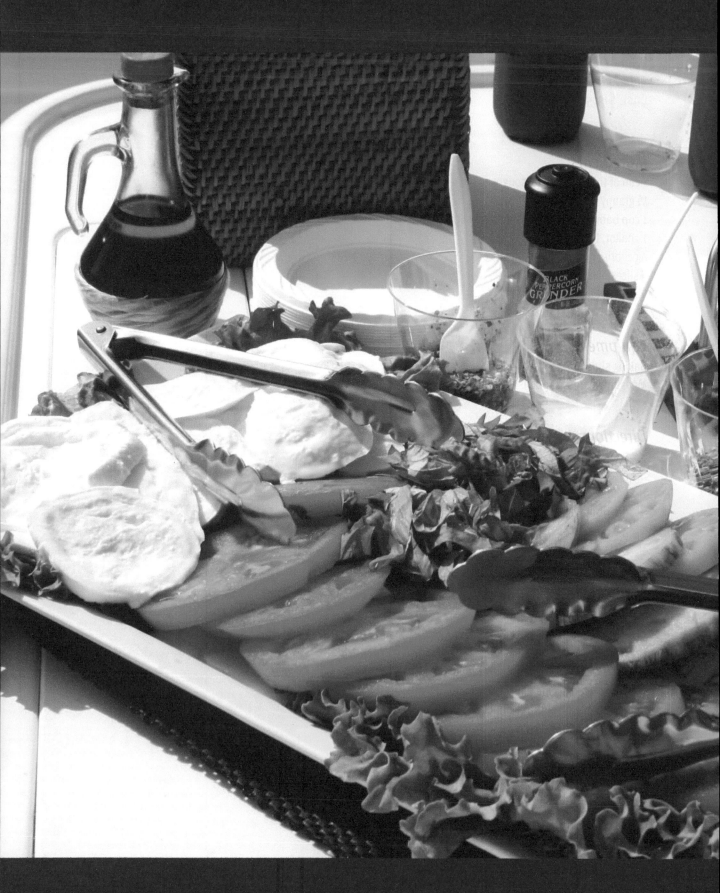

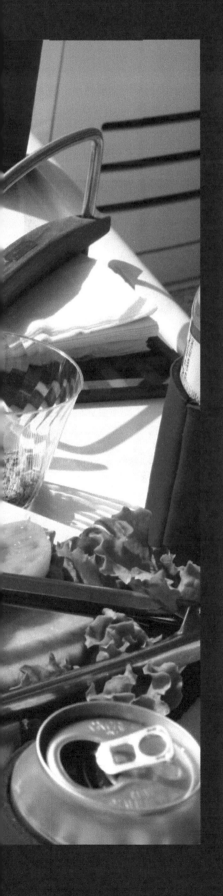

Tropical Salmon Salad

Delhi Chicken Salad

Cold Sesame Noodle Salad

Edamame Salad

Thai Papaya Salad

Sarimi Salad

Beachside Crab Salad with Mimosa Vinaigrette

Caesar Salad with Homemade Croutons and
    Parmesan Crisps

New Orleans Shrimp Salad

Mandarin Chicken Salad with Pomegranate
    Vinaigrette

Tijuana Taco Salad

TROPICAL SALMON SALAD

Who would have thought a gourmet fish salad could be so easy? Arugula is a spicy, peppery let-tuce and when you combine it with the richness of the salmon, saltiness of the cheese and sweet-ness of the mango you'll create a perfect harmony of flavors.

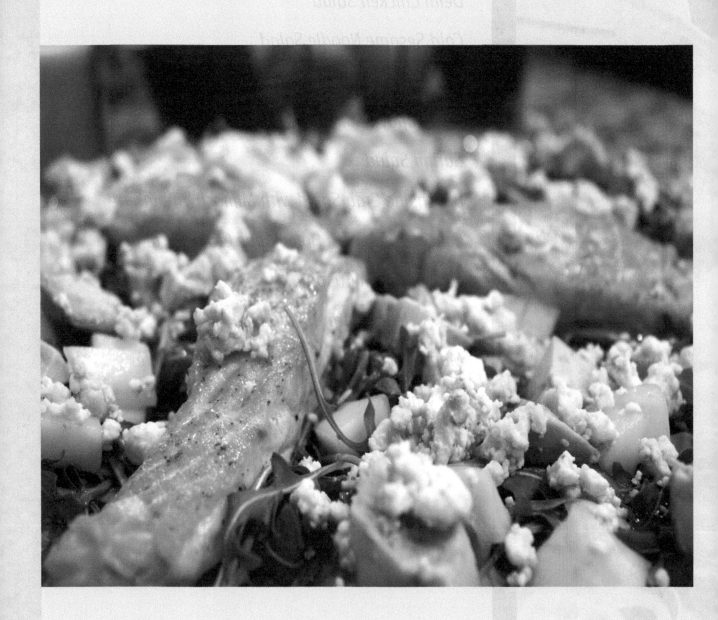

Servings: 4
Prep time: 10 minutes
Cooking time: 10 minutes
Cost: $19.49

Ingredients

1 lb. salmon (de-boned, skinless)
1 bunch baby Arugula (or prewashed bag or box)
Juice of 1 lemon
Juice of 1 lime
1 ripe mango
1 ripe avocado
4 oz. Gorgonzola
2 tablespoons vegetable oil (preferably canola)

Equipment

Sauté pan
Paring knife
Cutting board

Directions

1. Slice salmon on a cutting board with a paring knife into
    four equal sized pieces. Season both sides with salt
    and pepper; this is the best time to season raw fish
    or meat. Heat the pan over medium-high, allowing it
    to warm up before pouring in the vegetable oil.
    Gently place the salmon onto the hot pan.
    You should hear a sizzle when you do this — don't worry!
    This means the searing process will work properly.
    Sear on medium-high for 4 -5 minutes on each side for
    medium, 6 – 7 minutes on each side for well done.

2. Cube and cut the avocado and mango.
    Our general advice on cutting a mango is to work your
    way around the pit, slice around the pit and cut into
    cubes. To make sure your avocado stays fresh while
    you're working on the salmon, sprinkle it with lemon
    or lime juice.

3. On a large serving plate, place the avocado, mango,
    and Gorgonzola on a bed of arugula.
    Place the fish on the salad. Squeeze the juice of one
    fresh lime and one fresh lemon over the salad.
    No extra oil is necessary! It's light and delicious
    just like this.

DELHI CHICKEN SALAD

A taste of Southeast Asia on a hot summer day will give you a refreshing break from your internship, research, or tanning by the sun.
Great for picnics and tastes just as delicious the next day.

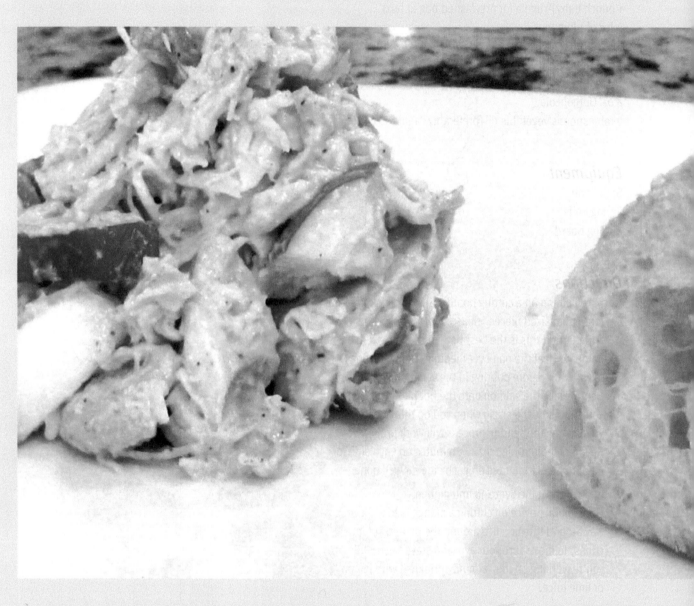

Servings: 4 – 6
Prep time: 5 minutes
Cooking time: 38 – 40 minutes
Cost: $6.77

Ingredients

1 ¼ lbs (about 20 oz.) boneless, skinless chicken breast
2 tablespoons olive oil
¼ cup lemon juice (juice of 1 lemon)
½ cup chicken stock (or water)
½ cup of golden raisins
½ fresh apple, sliced
½ cup mayonnaise
1 teaspoon of cumin
¼ teaspoon of salt (+ extra for seasoning chicken)
¼ teaspoon of pepper (+ extra for seasoning chicken)

Equipment

Mixing bowls
Sauté pan with cover
Cutting board & paring knife
Measuring cups & spoons

Directions

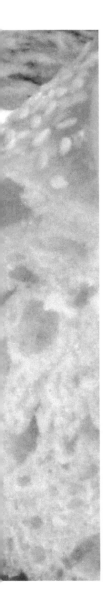

1. Heat a large sauté pan over medium-high heat. Once the pan is hot add 2 tablespoons of olive oil. Place the chicken breast in the pan and brown on both sides (about 4 minutes on each side). Make sure to season the chicken with salt and pepper on each side.

2. Once the chicken has browned add the lemon juice and chicken stock, cover the pan and cook for 30 minutes on medium-low.

3. Now you're ready for the making of the salad. Remove the chicken from the pan and cut into large chunks on a cutting board, then put the chicken in a mixing bowl. Add ½ cup of golden raisins and ½ fresh apple sliced into small chunks.

4. In a separate bowl, mix the mayonnaise with cumin, salt, and pepper. Add the mayonnaise mixture to the chicken and mix. Serve either on a bed of fresh salad greens or on some bread for a tasty sandwich!

COLD SESAME NOODLE SALAD

For those of you who can't get enough of that chilled peanut butter noodle taste from take-out Chinese restaurants, get ready to bring the flavors home. Our cold sesame noodle salad is quick and easy and will taste great for days afterwards.
The crunch of the carrots and the savory taste of the scallions add complexity to the peanut butter sauce. Grab some chopsticks and dig in!

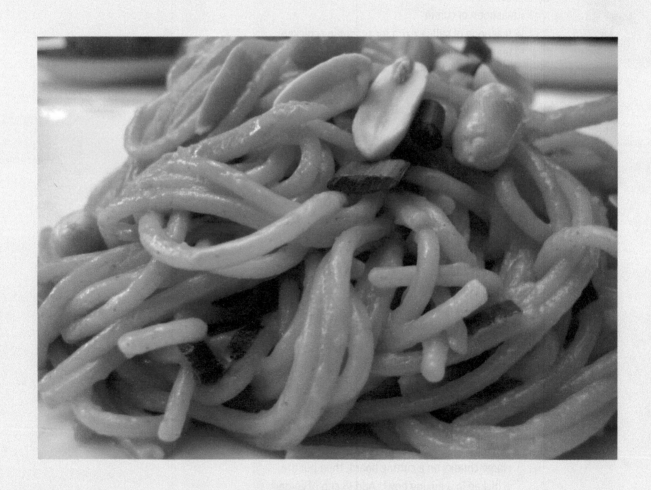

Servings: 6 - 8
Prep time: 15 minutes
Cooking time: 15 minutes
Cost: $7.30

Ingredients

1 lb. spaghetti
1 cup shredded carrots
3 green onions, chopped
½ cup peanuts (preferably unsalted)
1 cup peanut butter
¼ cup rice wine vinegar
¼ cup soy sauce
¼ cup honey
1 tablespoon sesame oil
½ teaspoon black pepper
1 cup vegetable broth (or water)

Equipment

Stock Pot /Pasta Pot
Cutting board with chopping/paring knife
Saucepan for making the peanut sauce
Grater for carrots (easiest to buy the carrots already shredded)
Measuring cups & spoons

Directions

1. Boil the pasta as per package directions. Remember to generously salt the water after it has begun to boil and before you pour in the raw pasta!
   After the pasta is done boiling, drain and return to the pot, add a teaspoon of sesame oil and a pinch of salt to the pot and mix thoroughly.

2. In a saucepan over medium-low heat, mix together the chicken stock, peanut butter, rice wine vinegar, soy sauce, honey, and pepper. Remember to spray your spoon with vegetable oil to help slide the honey off the spoon more smoothly. Stir occasionally for 8-10 minutes, until smooth and blended completely.

3. Add the peanut butter sauce to the pasta, mix well and refrigerate.

4. You can serve this dish warm, but we recommend refrigerating it for a couple of hours (until chilled) and serving it cold. Add the green onions and carrots after the pasta has chilled. Top each serving with a sprinkling of peanuts.

EDAMAME SALAD

You'll feel like you're at an upscale Japanese restaurant while eating this salad. It's elegant, simple, light, and healthy. Your friends will surely ask for the recipe.

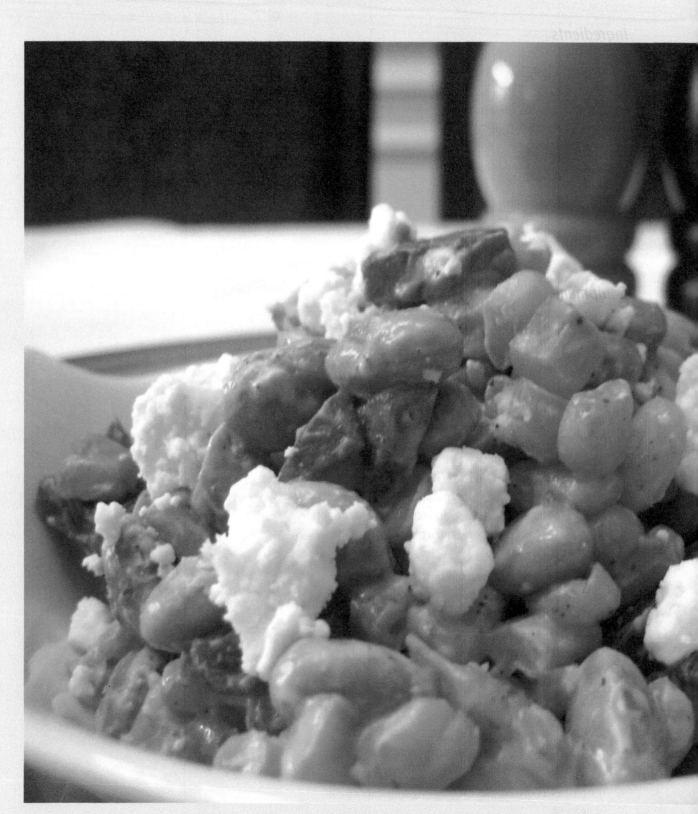

Servings: 4 - 6
Prep time: 5 minutes
Cooking time: 0 minutes
Cost: $6.61

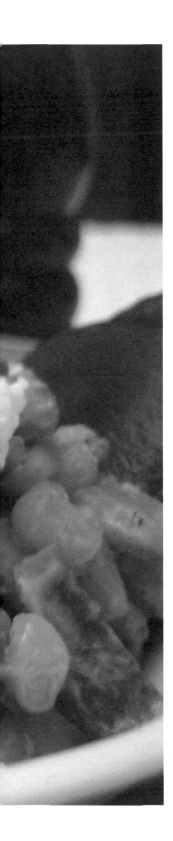

Ingredients
2 cups canned corn, drained
1 cup de-shelled edamames (fresh or frozen)
1 cup diced canned beets, drained
½ cup crumbled goat cheese
1 tablespoon rice wine vinegar
1 teaspoon salt
¼ teaspoon black pepper

Equipment
Mixing bowl
Measuring cups & spoons

Directions
Mix all ingredients together in a mixing bowl and serve with lettuce, as a side dish with a sandwich, or all by itself.

THAI PAPAYA SALAD

Papayas are loaded with vitamins and fiber. Buy them when they are half green and half yellow—at this stage they will be ready to eat in 1-2 days. If you can only find the green papayas they will take 5-6 days to be fully ripe.

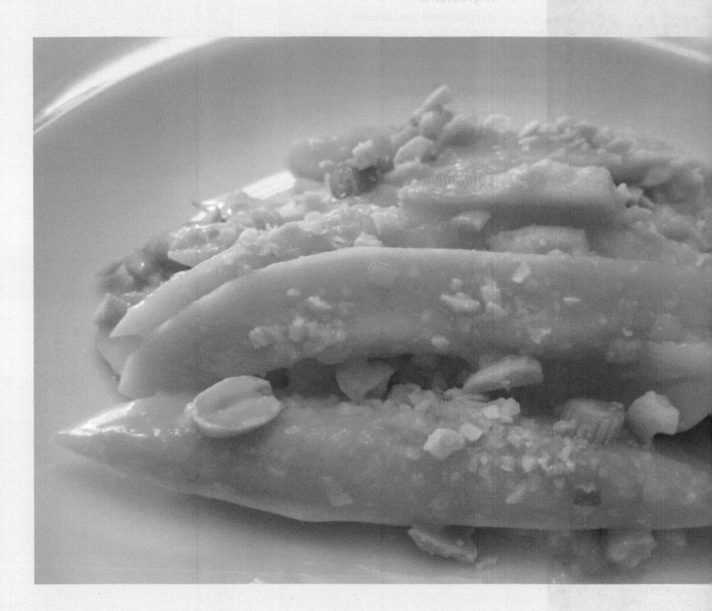

Servings: 4
Prep time: 10 minutes
Cooking time: 8 minutes
Cost: $6.38

Dressing Ingredients
½ cup coconut milk
2 sprigs lemongrass
½ teaspoon fresh ginger, grated
1 tablespoon sugar

Salad Ingredients
1 ripe papaya
½ cup fresh scallions, sliced
1 teaspoon lemon juice
1 tablespoon lime juice
¼ teaspoon salt
½ cup crushed unsalted peanuts

Equipment
Small saucepan
Mixing bowl
Measuring cups and spoons

Directions
1. Steep coconut milk, lemongrass, ginger, and sugar over medium-low in a small saucepan for 2 – 3 minutes, then turn down to low, stir, and steep on low for 5 minutes.

2. Be sure to remove the lemongrass and discard once the dressing has steeped sufficiently.

3. Wash papaya and peel carefully. Gently remove seeds with a spoon and discard. Slice the papaya into very thin slices. Put into a large mixing bowl and gently mix with lemon juice, lime juice, and salt. Add the scallions and crushed peanuts, pour the coconut milk dressing over, and gently mix until the salad is completely blended. Serve cold.

SARIMI SALAD

Sarimi is also known as imitation crab. But it's not fake fish, just fake crab.
It is actually made from Pollock (a fish). You are probably most familiar with it in
California rolls and the frozen fish sticks you loved as a kid.

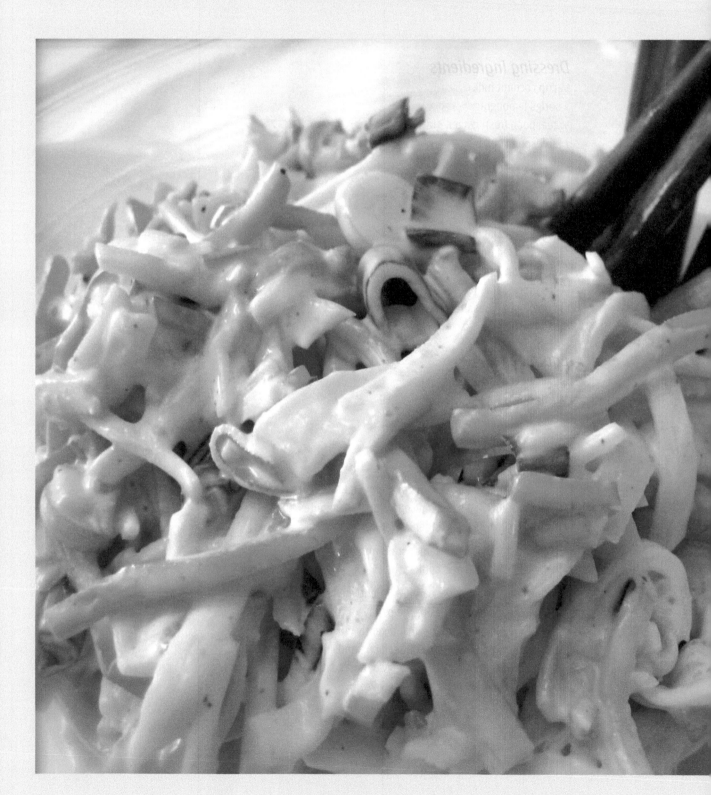

Servings: 4
Prep time: 10 minutes
Cooking time: 0 minutes
Cost: $3.99

Ingredients

1 x 8 oz. package sarimi*
2 green onions (scallions), sliced
½ cup shredded carrots
½ cup mayonnaise
2 tablespoons lemon juice
¼ teaspoon salt
1/8 teaspoon pepper

Equipment

Mixing bowl
Measuring cups & spoons

Directions

1. Pull long strips from the sarimi, much in the way
   you would pull strips of cheese from string cheese.
   Place in a large bowl. Add the green onions,
   carrots, and lemon juice. In a mixing bowl mix
   the mayonnaise, pepper, and salt. Add to the
   sarimi –onion mixture and toss to coat.

2. This can be served as a salad or as a sandwich
   on toasted bread with a piece of cheese.
   *NB: Sarimi, more commonly known as imitation
   crabmeat, can be found at your local grocery store.
   It comes in three varieties: flake, chunk, or leg.
   Select the 'leg.'

BEACHSIDE CRAB SALAD WITH MIMOSA VINAIGRETTE

You will feel like you're at the beach while eating this salad. It's light, healthy, and low-cal.

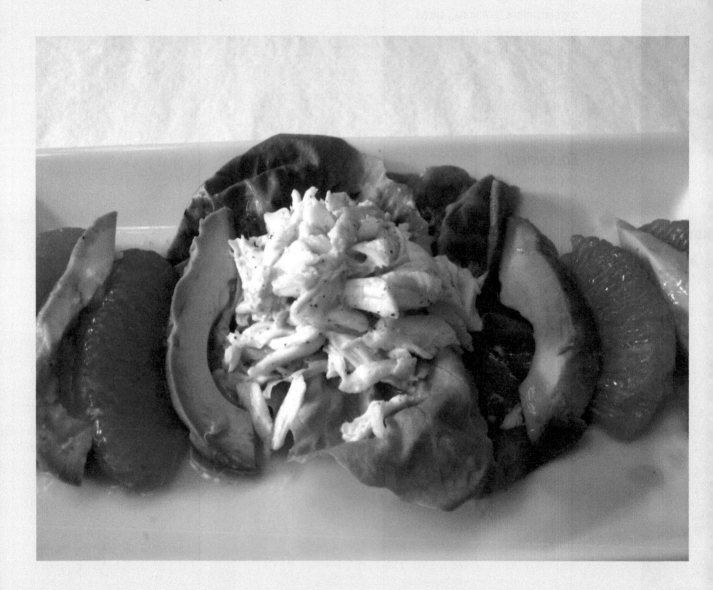

Servings: 4
Prep time: 10 minutes
Cooking time: 0 minutes
Cost: $10.72

Salad Ingredients
Butter lettuce
½ ripe avocado per plate
1 large grapefruit, 4 sections per plate

Crabmeat Ingredients
8 oz. lump crab meat
2 tablespoons lemon juice
1 tablespoon mayonnaise
½ teaspoon salt
¼ teaspoon pepper
Mimosa vinaigrette (below)

Mimosa Vinaigrette Ingredients
4 tablespoons olive oil
4 tablespoons orange juice
2 tablespoons champagne white wine vinegar
¼ teaspoon salt
½ teaspoon sugar
1/8 teaspoon black pepper

Equipment
Mixing bowls and spoons
Cutting board
Paring knife

Directions
1. Mix the crabmeat salad ingredients in a small mixing bowl.

2. To make the vinaigrette, we recommend using a measuring cup. A good ratio to stand by is 3:1 oil: vinegar, but we want a strong citrus taste so will be following a 2:1 ratio this time around. Whisk all the ingredients together.

3. Slice the avocado and grapefruit into wedges. Serve with the crabmeat and vinaigrette over a bed of butter lettuce for a refreshing and light lunch!

Caesar Salad With Homemade Croutons And Parmesan Crisps

Once you have made homemade croutons you will never buy the bagged version again!
Make the Parmesan crisps by themselves for an afternoon snack or a late night bite.

Servings: 6
Prep time: 10 minutes
Cooking time: 8 minutes
Cost: $8.88

Ingredients
1 box or package of prewashed romaine lettuce
1 loaf crusty bread (unsliced)
1 cup grated Parmesan cheese
¼ cup olive oil
1 tablespoon Mrs. Dash seasoning
Your favorite Caesar dressing
Shredded Parmesan for topping (optional)

Equipment
Baking sheet
Large sauté pan
Parchment paper (optional)

Directions
For the croutons: Slice the bread about ½ inch thick and
toast lightly in a 400 degree oven or in a toaster.
Cut the bread into cubes.
Plan for about 1 piece of bread per person.
Heat a large sauté pan over medium heat.
Once the pan is hot, add the oil, Mrs. Dash, and cubed bread
and sauté for 2-3 minutes.

For the Parmesan crisps: Mound 1 tablespoon of Parmesan
on a baking sheet and press down the center with the spoon.
Place in a 400 degree F oven for 5 minutes.

To make the salad: Place lettuce in a bowl, top with croutons,
Parmesan crisps, and drizzle with your favorite dressing.
Sprinkle with extra Parmesan, if desired.

NEW ORLEANS SHRIMP SALAD

This is our version of shrimp salad with a New Orleans twist. The cayenne pepper makes this dish a little spicy—if you like it spicier, add a full ½ teaspoon of cayenne. We think it's also wonderful on a toasted hoagie roll.

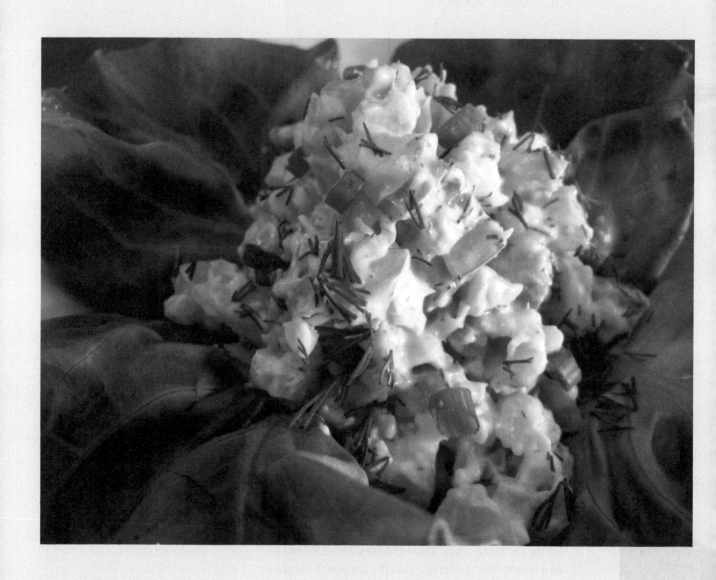

Servings: 4
Prep time: 5 minutes
Cooking time: 5 minutes
Cost: $11.78

Ingredients

1 pound of 21-25 shrimp (medium shrimp that comes 21-25
count to a pound)
½ cup mayonnaise
2 green onions (same as scallions), sliced
2 tablespoons fresh dill, chopped
2 tablespoons olive oil
4 tablespoons lemon juice, divided
1 teaspoon salt
½ teaspoon garlic powder
½ teaspoon onion powder
¼ teaspoon cayenne pepper

Equipment

Large sauté pan
Cutting board
Mixing bowls/spoons

Directions

1. Heat a large sauté pan over medium-high heat.
   Add the oil once the pan is hot. Then add the shrimp,
   2 tablespoons lemon juice, salt, garlic powder, onion
   powder, and cayenne pepper and cook for 5 minutes
   until the shrimp is cooked—it will turn pink once it is
   cooked. Do not over cook the shrimp—it will get tough
   and rubbery. Let cool and chop into small pieces.
   Set aside in a bowl.

2. In a mixing bowl mix the mayonnaise with the
   remaining 2 tablespoons of lemon juice.
   Add to the cooled shrimp. Fold in the dill and green
   onions and serve over lettuce. You can also serve
   this shrimp salad on a hoagie roll.

MANDARIN CHICKEN SALAD WITH POMEGRANATE VINAIGRETTE

Perfect for a light summer lunch or supper, this salad will wow your taste buds with bursts of fresh flavor. The cranberries are tender and succulent, the oranges sweet and light, the goat cheese sharp and tangy, and the chicken balances it all out for a healthy all-around meal. Feel free to eliminate the chicken for a delicious vegetarian salad.

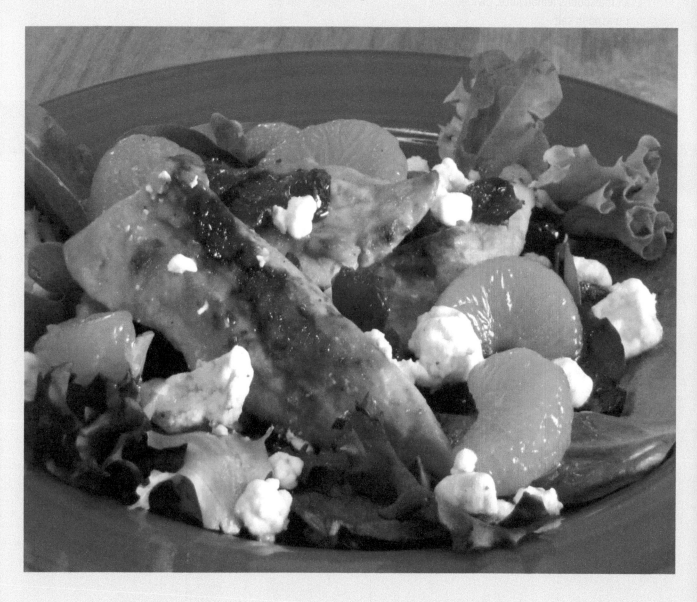

Servings: 4
Prep time: 5 minutes
Cooking time: 6 minutes
Cost: $14.73

Ingredients

1 pound chicken tenders
Juice of 1 lemon (1/4 cup)
3 tablespoons olive oil
2 tablespoons pomegranate juice
Salt & pepper
1 cup dried cranberries
4 or 5 oz. pack goat cheese crumbles
1 x 16 oz. can mandarin oranges
Spring lettuce mix

Vinaigrette Ingredients

¼ cup pomegranate juice
¼ cup rice wine vinegar
½ cup olive oil
1 tablespoon honey
1 tablespoon lemon juice
1 teaspoon mandarin juice (from can)

Equipment

1 large sauté pan
Measuring cups & spoons
Liquid measuring glass or bowl for making dressing

Directions

1. Heat a large sauté pan over medium heat. When the pan is warm add the olive oil and gently place the chicken tender strips into the pan. Sprinkle with salt and pepper.
   Add the juice of 1 lemon and 2 tablespoons pomegranate juice to the pan.
   Add the dried cranberries and sauté together with the chicken; this will marry all the flavors and add some plump juiciness to the cranberries. Since tenders are quick to cook, you will want to stand by the stove.
   6 to 8 minutes on each side should cook the chicken thoroughly — another way to tell is by noting when the middle begins to whiten from the bottom (at that point, you turn the strips over).

2. In a mixing bowl or glass measuring cup, combine the pomegranate juice, rice wine vinegar, honey, lemon juice, mandarin juice, and a pinch of salt and pepper.
   Whisk thoroughly. Next, add the olive oil in a slow stream whisking continuously.
   Don't worry if your vinaigrette separates a little— just be sure to mix vigorously before pouring it over the salad.

3. Prepare a couple handfuls of lettuce as a bed for each plate. Sprinkle with about ¼ cup of the crumbled goat cheese and 8 – 10 mandarin wedges.
   Place three to four tenders on each plate, sprinkle the cooked cranberries over the top, and drizzle with dressing.

   Secret tip: We like to tenderize the chicken by squeezing lemon juice over the chicken and letting it sit for 30 minutes.

TIJUANA TACO SALAD

We're taking you straight to Tijuana with this salad. It's rich, hearty, and soul satisfying. A south of the border comfort food. Hominy is a type of corn used frequently in Mexican cooking and is richer and thicker than traditional corn. It's readily available in the canned vegetable aisle or in the Mexican foods aisle. For a short cut you can use jarred salsa for the topping, but splurge for the fresh cilantro, it's so wonderful.

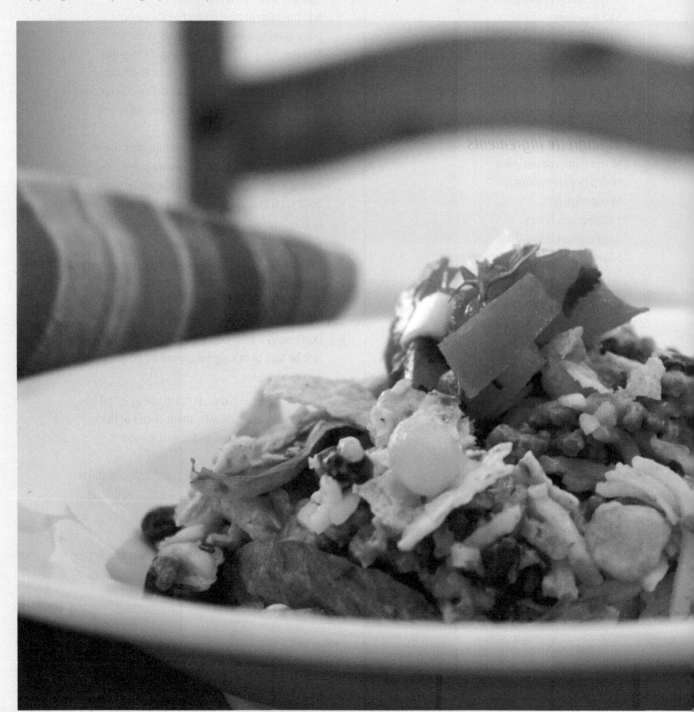

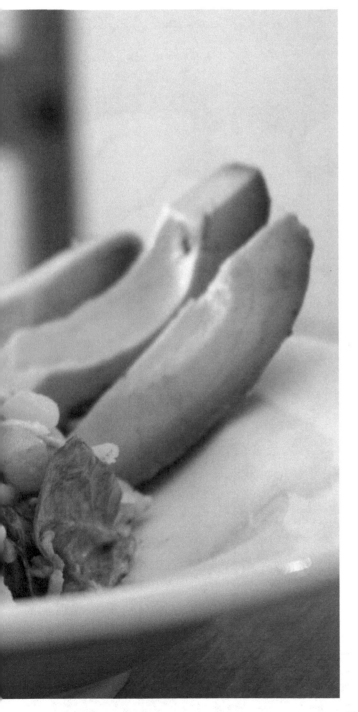

Ingredients

1 lb. ground beef
2 tablespoons oil
1 teaspoon salt
½ teaspoon ground black pepper
15 oz. can black beans, drained
15 oz. can hominy, drained
10 squirts of your favorite hot sauce
8 oz. bag Mexican cheese blend
2 handfuls of corn tortilla chips, crumbled
1 bag of lettuce of your choice
1 cup ranch dressing
1 avocado, sliced
Tomato salsa (recipe to follow)

Salsa Ingredients

1 large ripe tomato, diced
½ large red onion, diced
½ cup fresh cilantro, chopped
1 tablespoon lemon juice
1 tablespoon lime juice
½ teaspoon salt

Equipment

Large sauté pan
Mixing bowls
Measuring cups & spoons

Directions

1. First mix the salsa ingredients in a mixing bowl and set aside.

2. Heat a large sauté pan over medium heat and add 2 tablespoons oil and the ground beef, salt and pepper and cook over medium heat for 8-10 minutes until browned. Once the meat is cooked, add the black beans, hominy, hot sauce, and cook for another 5 minutes.
   Turn off heat and let cool.
   This is a room temperature salad. If you add hot meat/bean mixture to the lettuce it will wilt and the chips will get soggy.

3. To build your taco salad: Toss the lettuce with the beef & bean mixture, cheese, crumbled tortilla chips and ranch dressing. Top with homemade salsa and slices of avocado.

Servings: 6
Prep time: 5 minutes
Cooking time: 10 minutes
Cost: $10.62

6. Gourmet Sandwic and Burgers

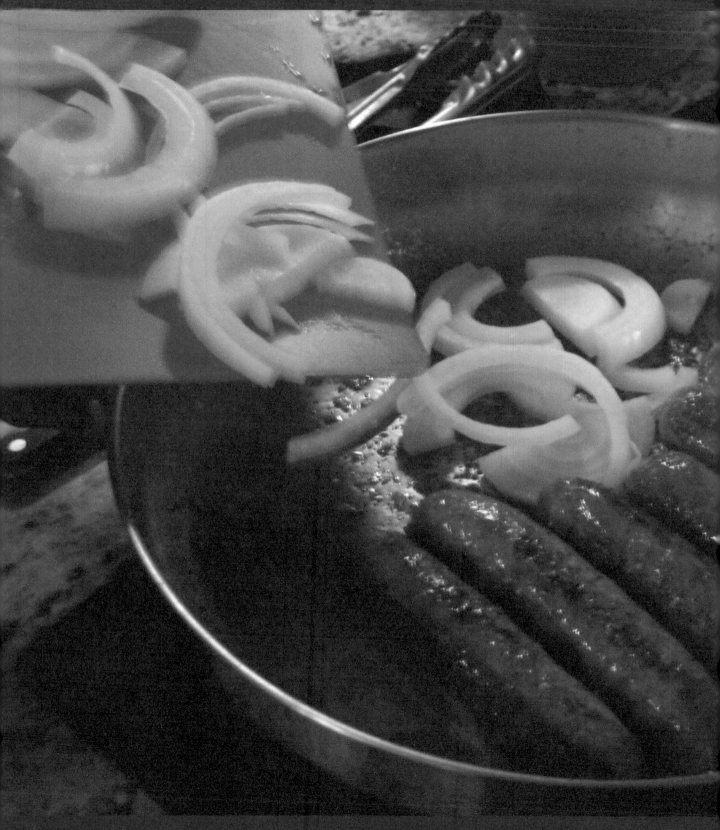

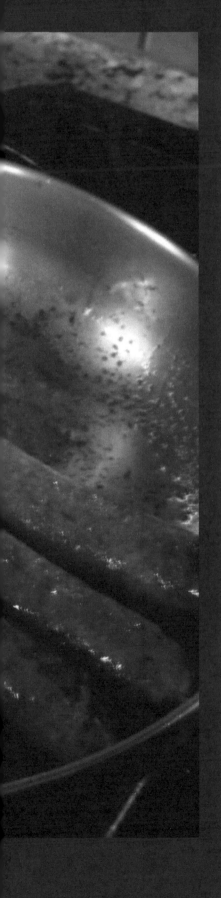

Thanksgiving Burger

Moroccan Burger with Mint Mayonnaise

Ham and Quattro Formaggi Panino

Crab Cake Burger

Mexican Burger with Mole Sauce

Panino Caprese

New Orleans Oyster Po' Boy Sandwich

Vienna Wiener Dogs

Portabella on a Portuguese Muffin

French Chicken Salad Sandwich

THANKSGIVING BURGER

Thanksgiving is a time for enjoying food. Why not enjoy the tastes particular to that holiday all year round? Our simple recipe gives you the taste and feeling of Thanksgiving any time of day or night.

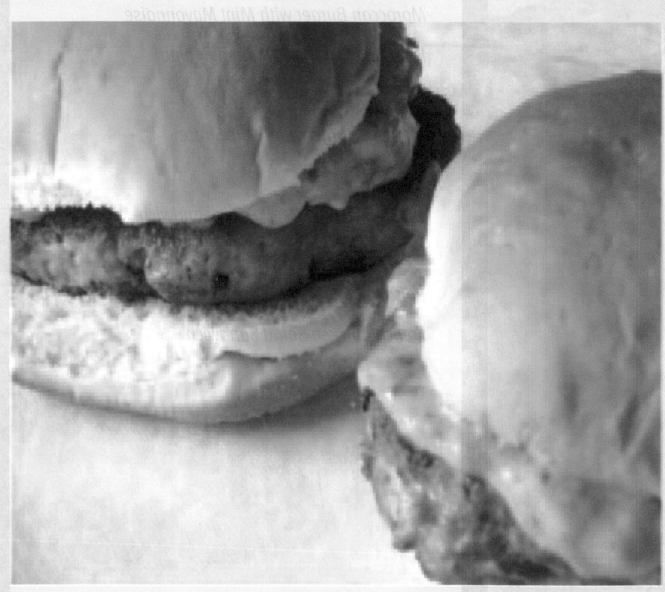

Servings: 6
Prep time: 10 minutes
Cooking time: 10 minutes per burger
Cost: $6.25

Burger ingredients

1 ¼ lbs. (20 oz.) of ground turkey
½ can of cut yams in syrup
½ cup of plain bread crumbs
1 fresh egg
¼ teaspoon of cinnamon
1 teaspoon of salt
½ teaspoon of pepper
1 tablespoon of unsalted butter

Aioli ingredients

2 heaping tablespoons of mayonnaise
3 heaping tablespoons of whole berry cranberry sauce
     (available in cans)

Equipment

Mixing bowl
Medium sauté pan

Directions

1. Empty the package of turkey into a large bowl and mix
   with the cut yams and breadcrumbs.
   Mash thoroughly with a fork (or even with your hands!).
   Crack a fresh egg into a small mixing bowl then add
   to the meat mixture (if you add the egg directly to
   the pan and there is any shell you may have to start
   over). Next mix in the cinnamon, salt, and pepper.

2. Set the stove on medium heat, and melt the butter in
   the sauté pan. Form the meat mixture into patties and
   cook for approximately 5 minutes on each side
   (until well done).

3. While the burgers are cooking, you can whip up a quick
   aioli that truly completes the Thanksgiving feeling.
   Mix the mayo and the cranberry sauce together in a
   bowl. Once the burgers are done, put them on a bun,
   slather with aioli, and enjoy a delicious holiday treat
   any time of the year!

MOROCCAN BURGER WITH MINT MAYONNAISE

A taste of the exotic in your every day. We've tried to pull together the flavors that remind us most of Moroccan cuisine for this original, easy to make burger.

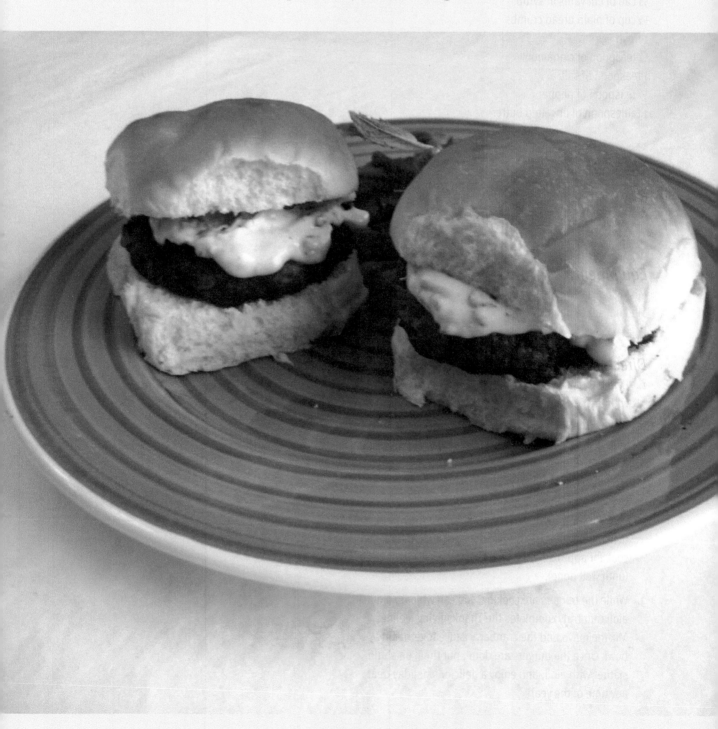

Servings: 4
Prep time: 10 minutes
Cooking time: 10 – 12 minutes
Cost: $7.64

Burger ingredients

1 lb. ground lamb meat
8 dried apricots (comes in 7 oz. bags), finely chopped
1/3 cup of golden raisins
1 teaspoon salt
½ teaspoon black pepper
1 tablespoon unsalted butter

Aioli ingredients

Leaves of 3 stalks of mint (about 6-8 leaves), finely chopped
½ cup mayonnaise
½ teaspoon cumin

Equipment

Large and small mixing bowls
Large sauté pan
Chopping knife

Directions

1. Finely chop the apricots. Put into a large mixing bowl with 1 lb. of ground lamb meat and the golden raisins. Add the salt and pepper. Mix together thoroughly. Heat a sauté pan over medium heat. Once the pan is hot add the butter. After forming the meat into patties cook for 5 – 6 minutes on each side.

2. To make the aioli, finely chop the leaves of 3 stalks of mint. Mix in a bowl with the mayonnaise and cumin. Slather on your burgers and enjoy while listening to some Arabic tunes!

Ham And Quattro Formaggi Panino

There aren't many words in the English language that can capture what a perfect combination of flavor and texture come in every bite with this panino twist on a classic deli sandwich. The sweet, smoky ham combined with the four layers of taste that come with the gooey melted cheese, the tangy bite of the pesto Dijon spread, the crunch of the crisp, golden bread—let's just say you will never think of ham and cheese the same way again.

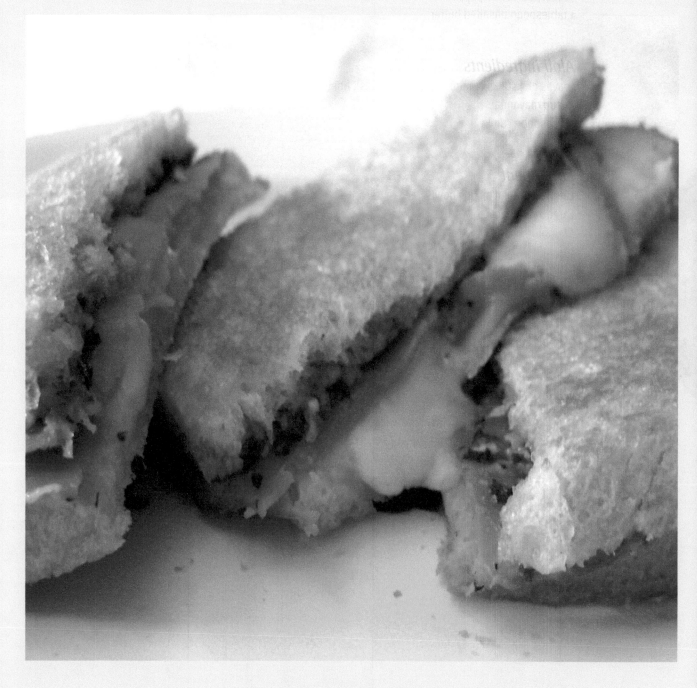

Servings: 4
Prep time: 10 minutes
Cooking time: 12 minutes
Cost: $14.77

Ingredients
Thinly sliced bread (preferably sourdough)
8 slices ham (2 per sandwich)
8 slices Munster cheese (2 per sandwich)
8 slices Provolone
8 slices Swiss
8 slices Mozzarella

Pesto Dijon Ingredients
1 cup basil leaves
2 tablespoons pine nuts
¼ cup olive oil
1 teaspoon Dijon mustard
2 teaspoons honey
½ cup grated Parmesan
¼ teaspoon of salt
¼ teaspoon of black pepper
1 teaspoon garlic paste

Equipment
Food processor
Spatula
Measuring cups & spoons
2 large sauté pans
Cans to weigh the sandwiches down

Directions
To make the pesto Dijon:
Mix the ingredients in a food processor until smooth.

To make the Panino:
Spread the pesto Dijon on the top piece of bread. Layer 2 pieces of each cheese* and 2 pieces of ham on the bottom piece of bread. Put the sandwich together and cook in a sauté pan over medium heat, about 3 minutes on each side, until browned. To press the sandwich down use another pan with filled cans as weights, pictured above.
Tip: Cut the cheese, if necessary, to distribute evenly over the bread.
* This may seem like a lot of cheese but because the sandwich is pressed, they all melt beautifully together

Homemade panino maker

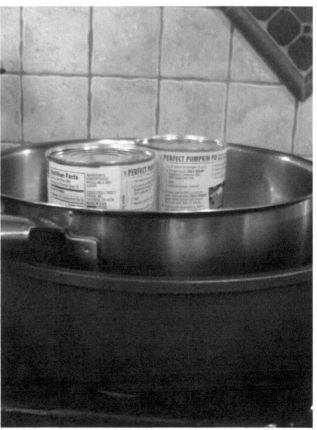

CRAB CAKE BURGER

*If you're longing for a taste of the shoreline, jet-set it to your local grocery store,
pick up some crab meat, and throw together our gourmet crab cake burgers!
Perfect for a summer dinner outdoors. Good crabmeat is expensive but at $ 4.75 per sandwich,
it's still cheaper to make it at home. The corn adds freshness and crunch.
Serve these light, healthy burgers with an arugula salad and iced tea.*

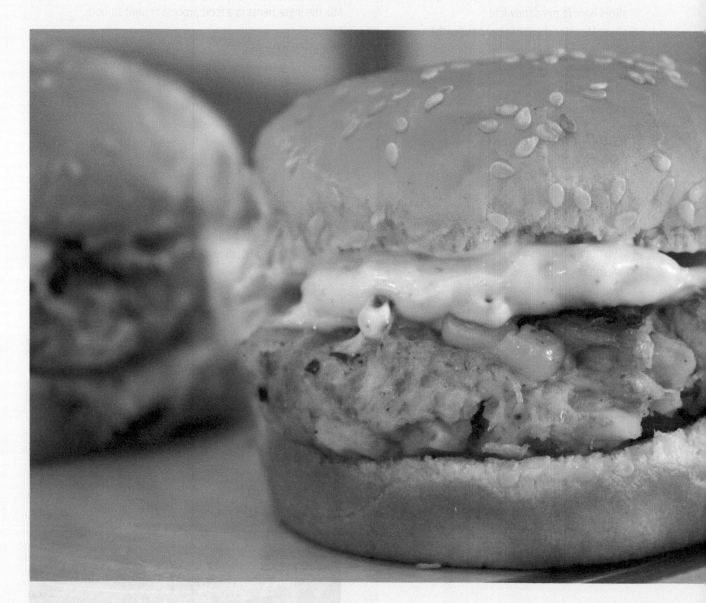

Servings: 6
Prep time: 15 minutes
Cooking time: 4 – 6 minutes
Cost: $28.50

Crab Patty Ingredients

16 oz. jumbo lump* crab meat
1/2 cup canned corn
1 cup breadcrumbs
1 egg, beaten
2 heaping tablespoons mayonnaise
2 tablespoons fresh tarragon, finely chopped
2 tablespoons lemon juice
1 teaspoon salt
½ teaspoon ground black pepper
1 teaspoon Old Bay seasoning (recommended to enhance flavor but not required)
2 tablespoons vegetable oil
2 tablespoons unsalted butter

Tartar sauce ingredients

3 heaping tablespoons of mayonnaise
2 heaping teaspoons of sweet relish
1 teaspoon of lemon juice
1/8 teaspoon cayenne pepper

Equipment

Mixing bowls
Sauté pan
Spatulas
Measuring cups & spoons
Whisk (or substitute with a spoon)

Directions

1. Roughly chop the tarragon. In a mixing bowl, combine the corn, breadcrumbs, egg, mayonnaise, tarragon, lemon juice, salt, and pepper, and mix thoroughly. Add the crabmeat and mix gently as to not break up the crab too much. Form the mixture into 6 patties.

2. Set the stove to medium heat. Melt 2 tablespoons of butter with the vegetable oil in the sauté pan and then place the patties in the pan. Cook for approximately two to three minutes on each side.

3. While the burgers are cooking, combine the ingredients for the tartar sauce in a bowl and mix thoroughly with a whisk or spoon. Slather either a Kaiser roll or regular hamburger bun with the tartar sauce. We also suggest serving the sandwich open-faced on a Portuguese roll or muffin. You can garnish with cucumber, lettuce, tomato, or whatever kind of refreshing vegetable suits your fancy.

*Jumbo lump crabmeat is the most expensive kind; less expensive varieties are also available and also very tasty.

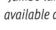

MEXICAN BURGER WITH MOLE SAUCE

Straight out of gourmet Tex-Mex cuisine, the Mexican Mole burger's got a wide range of tastes covered. From the juicy burger meat to the sweet and spiced mole sauce, you might not be able to eat just one!

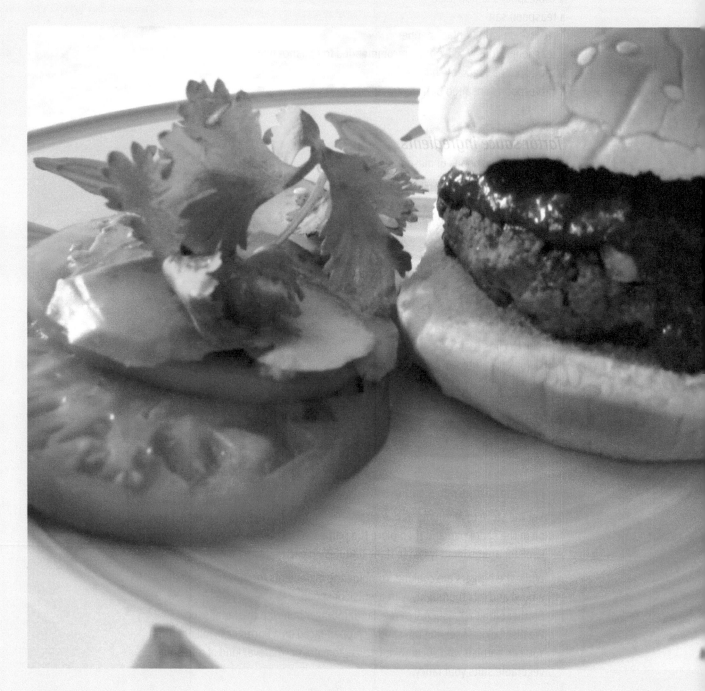

Servings: 4
Prep time: 25 minutes
Cook time: 25 minutes
Cost: $11.05

Burger Ingredients
1 lb. ground beef
1 teaspoon salt
½ teaspoon pepper
1/3 cup hominy (a type of corn)
2 tablespoons fresh chopped cilantro
2 tablespoons lime juice
2 tablespoons vegetable oil

Mole Sauce Ingredients
2 dried Ancho chilies
2 oz. bittersweet chocolate
1 onion, chopped
2 tablespoons vegetable oil
½ teaspoon cinnamon
½ teaspoon cumin
½ cup chicken stock
½ cup heavy cream or half and half
1 teaspoon salt

Equipment
Large sauté pan x 2
Small saucepan
Mixing bowls
Measuring cups & spoons

Directions
1. Rehydrate the Ancho chilies by placing them in a bowl with warm water for 15 minutes. Then removed the seeds and puree in a food processor.

2. Place the meat in a mixing bowl. Season with salt and pepper. Mix in the hominy, cilantro, and lime juice until blended. Do not overwork the meat.

3. Heat a sauté pan over medium heat and the oil once the pan is hot.
   Add the chopped onion and sauté for 3 minutes on medium heat.
   Add the chilies, cinnamon, cumin and cook for 5 minutes.
   Then add the stock and cream and cook for another 5 minutes. Let this mixture cool and puree in a food processor. Return the pureed mixture to a saucepan and melt the chocolate into the mixture over low heat.

4. Cook the burgers in another sauté pan with 2 tablespoons of oil on medium heat for about 6 minutes per side. Place the finished burger on a bun and cover with the chocolate mole sauce. Serve with freshly sliced avocado and tomato on the side or on top of the burger.
   You'll definitely have leftover mole, so refrigerate and use as a sauce for chicken the next day!

PANINO CAPRESE

Caprese salad on a sandwich? Of course. Why not! We've taken the classic Italian salad and created a unique taste sensation that will have your friends begging for another.

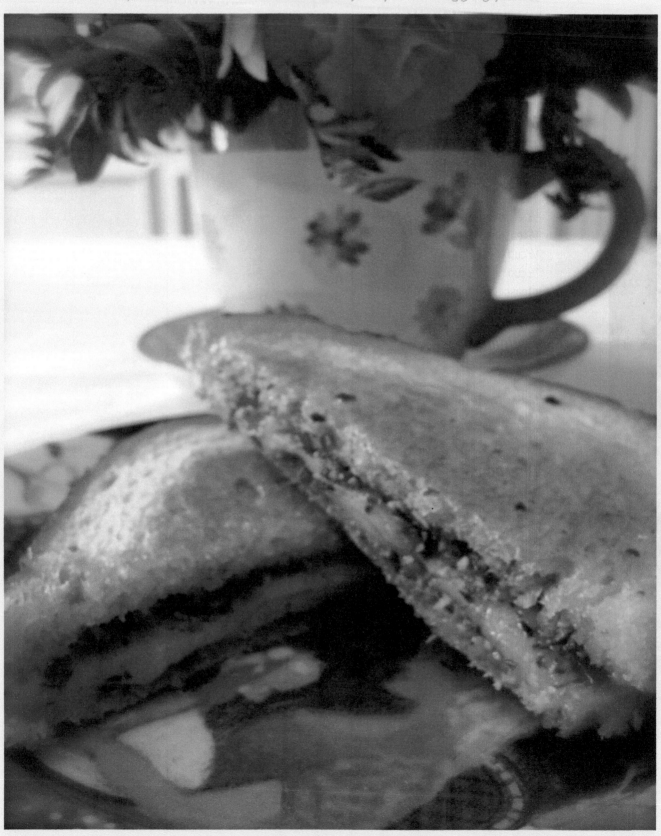

Servings: 4
Prep time: 10 minutes
Cooking time: 4 minutes
Cost: $15.41

Ingredients
8 slices Mozzarella (2 per sandwich)
Thinly sliced bread (preferably sourdough)
2 tablespoons olive oil
Sundried tomato pesto (see below)

Sundried Tomato Pesto Ingredients
2 cups basil leaves
4 tablespoons pine nuts
½ cup olive oil
½ cup grated Parmesan
½ teaspoon of pepper
2 teaspoons garlic paste
4 sundried tomatoes

Equipment
Food processor
Sauté pan (plus a smaller sauté pan and 2 cans of vegetables
or beans to make a homemade panino maker)

Directions
1. In a food processor, blend the basil, pine nuts, olive oil,
   Parmesan, and tomatoes. Then add the garlic paste and
   pepper and blend until the tomatoes are in small bits
   and the mixture has taken on a pesto-like texture.

2. Heat a large sauté pan over medium-high and add 2
   tablespoons of olive oil. On the counter, spread the
   pesto over both inner sides of the bread generously,
   then place one slice of mozzarella cheese on each side.
   Close the sandwich and place it in the heated sauté pan.
   Cook for about 2 minutes on one side (until golden brown),
   then flip the sandwich over with a spatula and weigh
   down with a heavy pan containing two cans (see picture of
   homemade panino maker in the Ham and Quattro Formaggi
   Panino recipe).
   Sear for another two minutes, then remove and serve.

NEW ORLEANS OYSTER PO' BOY SANDWICH

Bring a real taste of the Bayou home to your friends with our take on the classic oyster po' boy. Succulent oysters, fried golden and exploding with juices, combined with our spicy tartar sauce, will transport you to the waterfront and make you want to stay. Great for company any time of year, from chilly autumn nights to lazy summer afternoons.

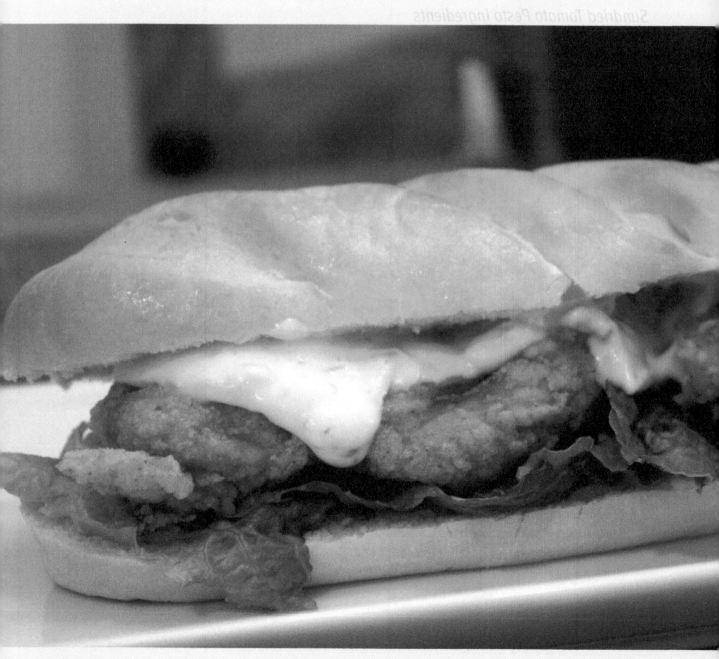

Ingredients

Oysters (2 packages, about 6 oysters per sandwich)
2 cups fish fry mix (comes in boxes)
1 cup whole milk or buttermilk
10 squirts of your favorite hot sauce
Vegetable oil for frying
Lettuce
Hoagie rolls (4)
Tartar sauce (see below)

Servings: 4
Prep time: 5 minutes
Cooking time: 15 minutes
Cost: $30.05

Tartar sauce ingredients

3 heaping tablespoons of mayo
2 heaping teaspoons of sweet relish
1 teaspoon of lemon juice
1/8 teaspoon cayenne pepper
Equipment
Large, deep saucepan for frying
Candy thermometer
Mixing bowls
Measuring cups & spoons

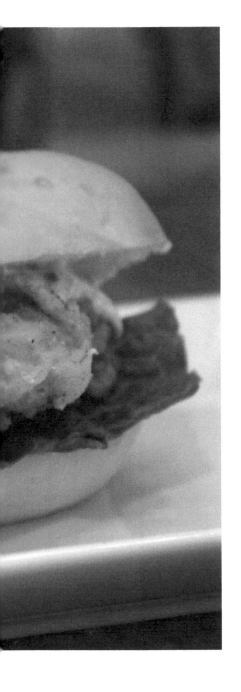

Directions

1. In a mixing bowl, combine and mix the ingredients for the tartar sauce. You can set this aside or put it in the fridge up to a day in advance of your cooking.

2. Fill the saucepan with oil—about half way up. (Do not fill higher because when you heat oil then add food, the oil will rise and can spill over and cause a fire.) Heat the oil over medium heat for about 5 minutes—the temperature should be 350 degrees F.
    If you have a candy thermometer, you can place it in the oil and leave it there to monitor your temperature.

3. In a mixing bowl add together the buttermilk and hot sauce.
    Pour the fish fry mixture into a separate bowl and line up the bowls next to the stove. Drain the oysters.

4. Dip the oysters first in the buttermilk, then into the fish fry, and then slowly place (do not drop) them into the hot oil.
    Turn the oysters once with tongs about halfway through the frying process (after about 2 minutes).
    Do not overcrowd the pan with oysters—they will not cook properly.
    It should take about 4 minutes to cook each batch of oysters.
    You will need to cook 3 to 4 batches depending on the size of your pan.
    Remove them and place on a paper towel to drain excess oil.

5. Sprinkle with salt and serve with iceberg lettuce and our homemade tartar sauce on a large roll (preferably one with a slit down the side).

VIENNA WIENER DOGS

Talk about your gourmet hot dog! We wanted to do a classic hot dog with a twist, so we're calling on the rich flavors of bratwurst sausage and sautéed onions. Our homemade tangy relish is really a union of the three staple hot dog condiments— ketchup, mustard, and relish. So simple but so special, you may never eat a normal hot dog again!

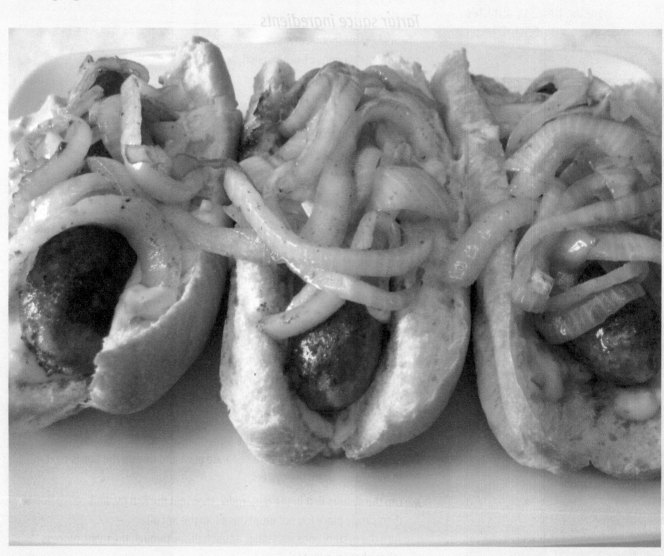

Servings: 4
Prep time: 5 minutes
Cooking time: 10 minutes
Cost: $7.75

Ingredients

4 bratwurst sausages, uncooked
4 large hot dog buns
1 large white onion, sliced
1 teaspoon onion powder
1 teaspoon garlic powder
1 tablespoon olive oil

Relish Ingredients

1/3 cup mayonnaise
3 tablespoons Dijon mustard
3 heaping tablespoons sweet relish
1 tablespoon ketchup

Equipment

Large sauté pan
Mixing bowl
Measuring cups & spoons

Directions

1. Heat a sauté pan over medium-low.
   Once the pan is hot add the olive oil.
   Place the sausages in the pan along with the onions, onion powder, and garlic powder, making sure that all ingredients are covered with the powders to attain maximal flavor.

2. Cook about 3 minutes per side, turning each sausage three times in total to ensure that the meat is cooked thoroughly. (About 10 minutes of cooking.)

3. While the onions and sausages are cooking, mix the relish ingredients thoroughly in a bowl.

4. Toast the buns until they brown.

5. Lather the buns with generous portions of the relish, top with the sausage and onions, and serve.

PORTABELLA ON A PORTUGUESE MUFFIN

Not your average lunchtime fare! We've created an elegantly simple sandwich with distinct flavors that really epitomize light gourmet eating. The creamy, herb-flavored Boursin cheese works well with the sweet tang of balsamic vinegar, and the mushrooms burst with tender juiciness in every bite. You may have trouble eating just one! If you cannot find Portuguese muffins in your local market, you can purchase them on-line from Amaral's in Fall River, Massachusetts at www.amaralsbakery.com.

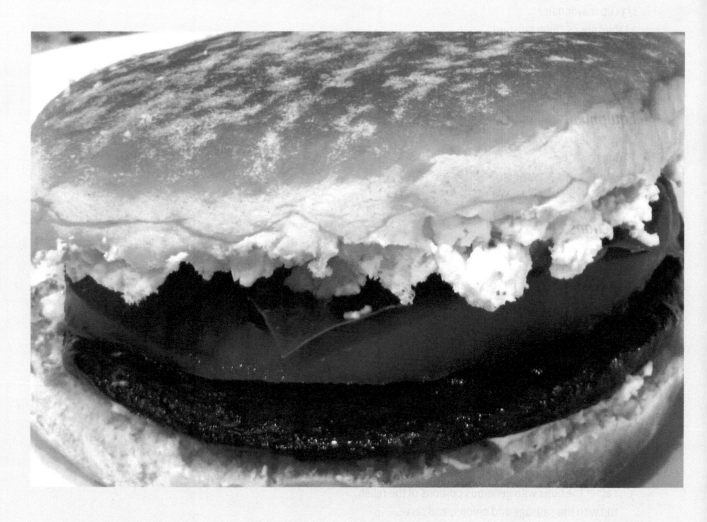

Servings: 4
Prep time: 5 minutes
Cooking time: 10 minutes
Cost: $15.71

Ingredients
1 package Boursin cheese (comes in 5.2 oz packages)
4 large portabella mushroom caps, whole
    (comes loose or in 6 oz packs of 2 caps)
4 slices of a large, ripe tomato (1 per sandwich)
Fresh basil leaves (3 per sandwich)
4 Portuguese muffins or sandwich-sized English muffins (plain)

Marinade Ingredients
½ cup balsamic vinegar
½ cup olive oil
1 tablespoon pomegranate juice
½ teaspoon ground black pepper

Equipment
Marinating dish (large enough to fit 4 mushroom caps)
Large sauté pan
Mixing bowl
Measuring cups & spoons

Directions
1. Before cooking the mushrooms, marinate them in a
   large Tupperware or dish with the balsamic vinegar,
   olive oil, pomegranate juice, and black pepper for about
   30 minutes, until the mushrooms have soaked in the
   juices thoroughly.
   Turn them a couple of times while they are marinating.

2. Heat a large sauté pan over medium heat.
   Add the mushrooms and sauté for 4 to 5 minutes per side.

3. While the mushrooms are cooking, spread Boursin on
   each side of the sandwich muffins.
   Place the portabella on the muffin, add the tomato slice,
   top with basil leaves, and cover with the other half of
   the muffin for a gushing blast of flavor.

FRENCH CHICKEN SALAD SANDWICH

*A couple of secret ingredients make this chicken salad sandwich u
thousand times better than the store-bought version — cumin and tarragon
(shh, don't tell your friends—make them try and guess).*

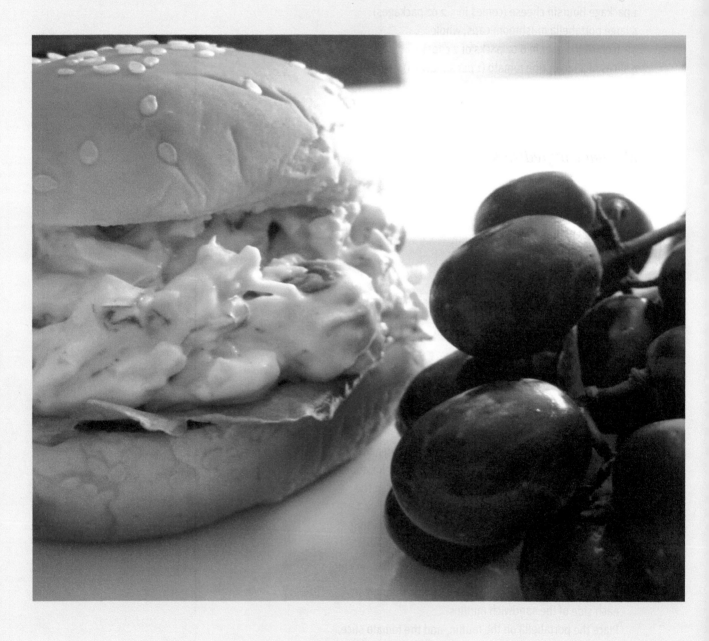

Servings: 4
Prep time: 10 minutes
Cooking time: 4 minutes
Cost: $11.41

Ingredients

1 pound package boneless, skinless chicken breast
2 tablespoons unsalted butter
½ cup water or chicken broth
2 tablespoons Dijon mustard
½ cup seedless grapes, halved
4 pieces of butter lettuce or 1 cup bagged lettuce
4 Kaiser rolls
Tarragon mayonnaise (see below)

Tarragon Mayonnaise

½ cup mayonnaise
½ cup sour cream
2 tablespoons chopped fresh tarragon
1 tablespoon lemon zest
1 tablespoon lemon juice
¼ teaspoon cumin
½ teaspoon salt
¼ teaspoon ground black pepper

Equipment

Medium sized sauté pan 9 to 10 inches
Chopping/paring knife
Measuring cups/spoons
Zester
Small and medium mixing bowls

Directions

1. Heat a sauté pan over medium heat. Once the pan is hot melt the
    butter in the pan and add the chicken. Cook on each side for about 2 minutes.
    Add the Dijon and the water and turn the heat down to medium-low.
    Cover and simmer for 30 minutes. Let cool.
    Cut into small pieces and place in a medium-size mixing bowl.
    Add the halved grapes.

2. To make the tarragon mayonnaise: in a small mixing bowl, mix the mayonnaise,
    sour cream, tarragon, lemon juice and zest, cumin, salt and pepper.
    Add the tarragon mayonnaise to the chicken and grapes and mix well.

3. Place a piece of lettuce on the bottom half of a Kaiser roll (or your favorite bread)
    top with chicken salad and serve with a side of fresh fruit or green salad.

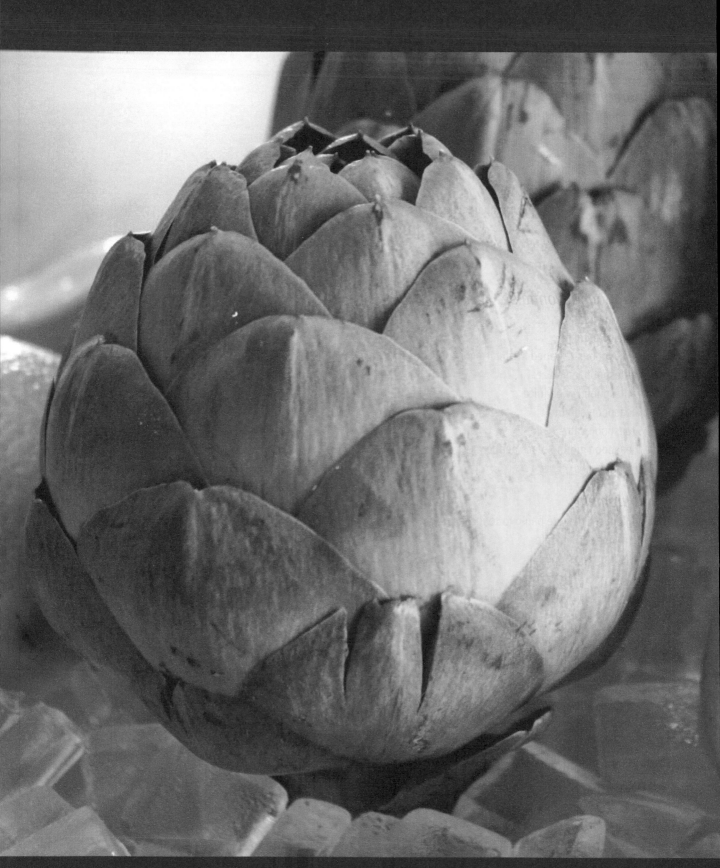

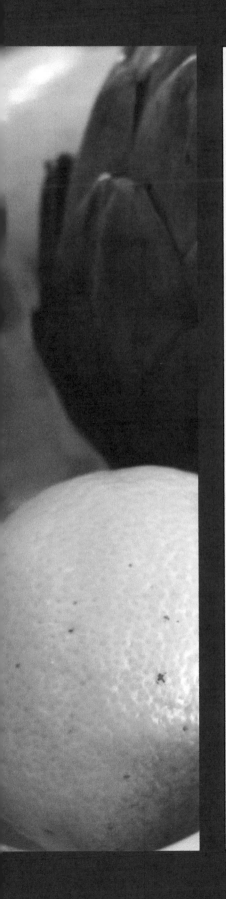

Refreshing Farfalle

Lemon Pasta

Pomegranate Pasta

Gorgonzola Portabella Penne

Spaghetti with Keftethes and Garlic Bread

New Orleans Andouille Pappardelle

Moroccan Stuffed Shells with Curried Béchamel

Artichoke Pesto Alfredo

Cheese Tortellini with Pumpkin and Fried Sage

REFRESHING FARFALLE

This light, healthy pasta dish is great for lunch on a summer day.
It's also wonderful cold for a midnight snack. And perhaps most importantly,
you can make this in under 15 minutes.

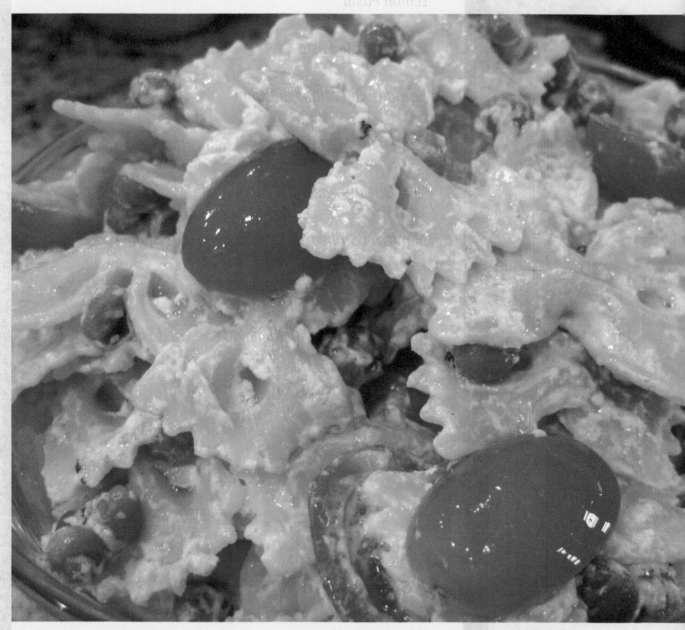

Servings: 6 - 8
Prep time: 5 minutes
Cooking time: 12 minutes
Cost: $ 12.75

Ingredients
1 pound farfalle pasta (bowtie)
2 cups frozen or canned peas
2 cups cherry or grape tomatoes, halved
2 cups your favorite Italian dressing
1 cup crumbled goat cheese

Equipment
Pasta pot
Colander
Measuring cups
Small saucepan (if using frozen peas)

Directions
1. Cook pasta according to the box directions.
   Drain and add the Italian dressing. Mix well.

2. If using frozen peas, cook over medium heat in a
   small saucepan for 5 minutes in 2-3 inches of water.
   Drain and add to the pasta.
   If you are using canned peas, drain and add directly
   to the pasta.

3. Add the tomatoes and goat cheese and mix.

4. Serve warm, room temperature, or cold.

LEMON PASTA

*Here's a great recipe for using the elements you have on hand
to create a quick meal for your gourmet friends.*

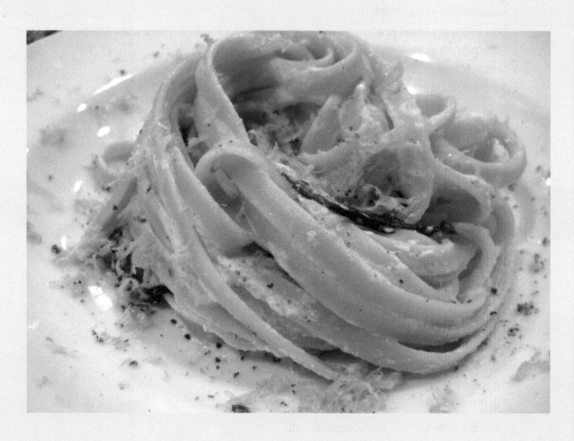

Servings: 4 - 6
Prep time: 10 minutes
Cooking time: 15 minutes
Cost: $8.56

Ingredients

16 oz. fettuccini
1 head of radicchio, sliced in strips
¾ cup grated Parmesan
½ teaspoon black pepper
2 tablespoons salt + 1 teaspoon
2½ cups cream or half and half
½ cup lemon juice (the juice of 2 lemons)
2 tablespoons unsalted butter
Freshly grated nutmeg (optional)
Lemon zest (optional)

Equipment

Sauté pan
Pasta pot
Colander
Measuring cups & spoons

Directions

1. Begin to cook the fettuccini as per the directions on the package.
   When the water comes to a boil, add 2 tablespoons salt to the pot.
   While the pasta is boiling, quarter 1 small head of radicchio, making
   sure to cut out and discard the core.
   Slice the radicchio into thin strips.

2. Sauté the radicchio in butter, over medium-low heat for 3 -5 minutes,
   until wilted. Leave the stove on a medium-low heat.
   Add the cream, grated Parmesan, pepper, and 1 teaspoon salt, and let
   the sauce reduce over 8-10 minutes while the pasta is cooking,

3. Drain the pasta and reserve the pasta water in case the sauce needs
   to be thinned out.
   When the pasta is done, add it to the sauté pan with the radicchio-cream
   sauce, add the lemon juice and toss to coat all the pasta with sauce.
   To add a little more flavor, sprinkle some fresh lemon zest and nutmeg
   over each individual dish.

POMEGRANATE PASTA

Pomegranate is a wonderfully versatile fruit and very in vogue today. We use the bottled juice in this recipe. They are touted to have anti-cancer and heart healthy effects. They're packed with antioxidants, vitamin C, and fiber, and are low in calories. We like to use cavatappi pasta in this recipe, cavatappi means corkscrew in Italian. Any short pasta with ridges to hold the sauce will work with this refreshing sauce.

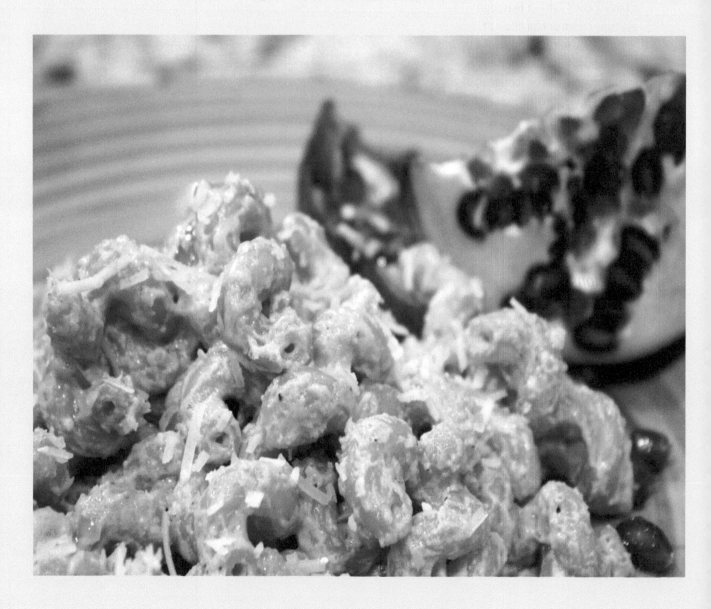

Servings 6 - 8
Prep time: 4 minutes
Cooking time: 15 minutes
Cost: $11.57

Ingredients
1 lb Cavatappi pasta (any short pasta with ridges will do)
1 cup goat cheese
4 oz. white cheddar cheese, cut into thin slices for easy melting,
    or grated with a box grater
½ cup Parmesan
1 cup pomegranate juice
2 tablespoons flour
2 tablespoons oil
1 cup cream
2 shallots, finely chopped
½ teaspoon ground black pepper
2 tablespoons salt (for salting the pasta water)

Equipment
Pasta pot
Medium sauté pan
Measuring cups & spoons
Box grater (optional)

Directions
1. Cook the pasta as per package directions.
    Be sure to salt the water after it comes to a boil!

2. In a sauté pan, cook the shallots in the oil over medium-low
    heat until soft, about 3-4 minutes.
    Next add the flour and stir continuously for about 1 minute
    until you have a blond color (the flour acts to thicken the sauce).

3. Add the pomegranate juice, cream, and cheeses, salt,
    and pepper to the sauté pan and increase the heat to
    medium-high until it comes to a boil, once it comes to a boil
    reduce the heat to medium-low and cook for 8-10 minutes
    until the cheese melts and the sauce is thick, smooth,
    and creamy.
    Add cooked pasta, sprinkle with Parmesan, stir and serve.

GORGONZOLA PORTABELLA PENNE

As you can see, we love Gorgonzola! Especially when paired with portabella mushrooms and figs. This is elegant comfort food.

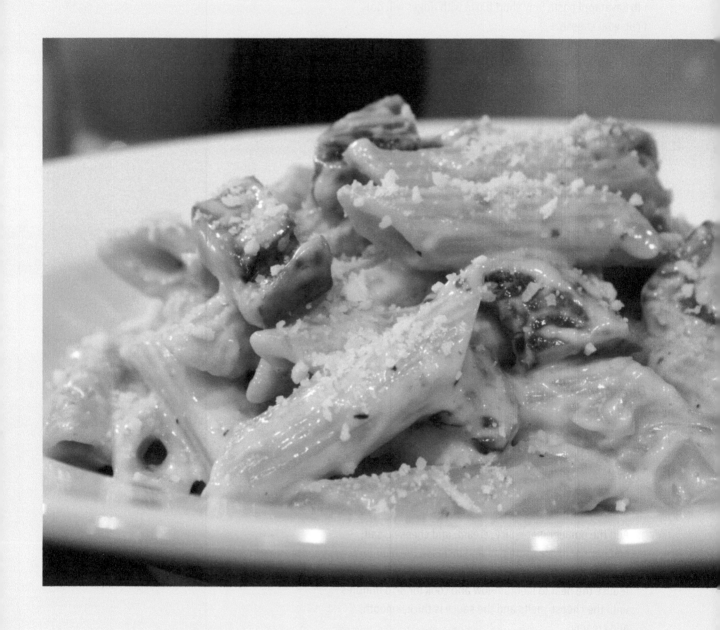

Servings: 6 - 8
Prep time: 5 minutes
Cooking time: 15 minutes
Cost: $14.60

Ingredients
1 lb. penne pasta
8 oz. gorgonzola cheese
6 oz. portabella mushrooms
½ large or 1 small yellow onion, finely chopped
¼ cup Parmesan cheese
2 cups cream or half and half
4 tablespoons fig spread (comes in jars)
2 tablespoons unsalted butter
2 tablespoons olive oil
1 teaspoon salt (+ 2 tablespoons for salting the pasta water)
½ teaspoon black pepper

Equipment
Pasta Pot
Cutting Board
Sauté pan
Measuring cups & spoons

Directions
1. Boil the pasta as per package directions.
   Be sure to salt the water after it comes to a boil!

2. Chop the mushrooms roughly and the onion finely
   on a cutting board, then add to a large sauté pan with
   olive oil, butter, salt, and pepper.
   Sauté for 5 – 8 minutes over medium-high heat.

3. Add the cream, Gorgonzola, Parmesan, and fig spread
   let the sauce come to a boil. Once the sauce is boiling
   turn down the heat to medium-low and simmer for
   6 - 8 minutes until the sauce thickens.

4. Toss in the cooked pasta and sprinkle with Parmesan
   and serve warm.

SPAGHETTI WITH KEFTEDES AND GARLIC BREAD

This is the way Ellen's Yia-Yia (Yia-Yia is Greek for grandmother) used to make spaghetti with meatballs (Keftedes). She always added a lot of butter to all of her recipes. The brown butter here gives the spaghetti a very rich, nutty flavor.

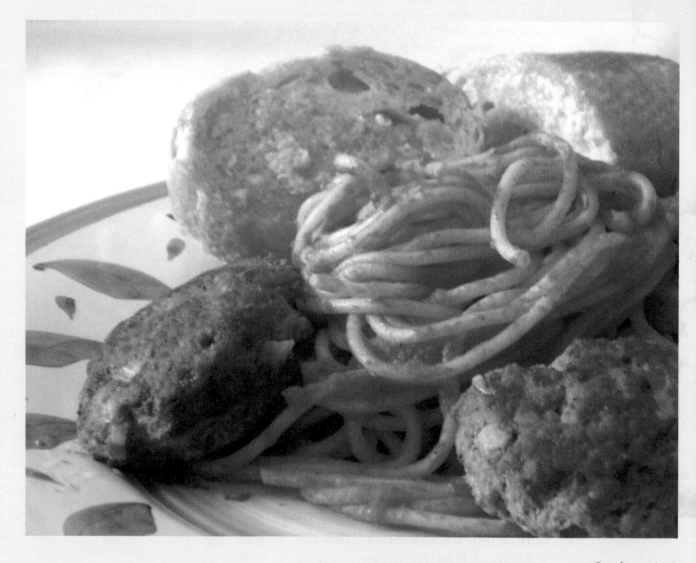

Servings: 6 - 8
Prep time: 5 minutes
Cooking time: 1 hour
Cost: $13.51

Ingredients

1 lb. spaghetti
1 stick unsalted butter (for brown butter sauce)
Tomato sauce (see below)
Keftedes (see below)
Garlic bread (see below)

Garlic Bread Ingredients

1 loaf French bread
2 tablespoons garlic paste (comes in tubes)
½ cup olive oil
Salt and pepper to taste

Tomato Sauce Ingredients

2 x 28 oz. cans crushed tomatoes
¼ cup tomato paste (comes in cans or tubes)
2 tablespoons sugar
1 teaspoon salt
½ teaspoon ground black pepper

Keftedes Ingredients

1 lb ground beef
2 slices toasted white bread
1 egg, beaten
¾ cup water
¼ large yellow onion, finely chopped (about ½ cup)
½ teaspoon dried oregano (can use fresh if you have it)
1 teaspoon dried parsley (can use fresh if you have it)
2 tablespoons unsalted butter
2 tablespoons canola oil
½ teaspoon salt
¼ teaspoon black pepper

Equipment

Large sauté pan
Pasta pot
Baking sheet
Mixing bowls
Measuring cups & spoons
Aluminum foil
Pastry brush (optional)

Directions

1. Heat the sauce ingredients in a large saucepan over low heat for about 1 hour.

2. Cook the pasta according to the package directions.

3. To make the garlic bread: Preheat the oven to 350 degrees F. Slice the bread in half, lengthwise. Mix the olive oil and the garlic paste in a small mixing bowl. Spread the garlic-oil mixture over each half of the bread, sprinkle with salt and pepper, and bake for 20 minutes.

4. To make the keftedes: Toast two slices of white bread lightly, moisten with the water and place in a bowl with the beaten egg, chopped onion and other ingredients, and thoroughly blend.
At this point, add the raw ground beef.
Once mixed, shape the meat into small patties with flattened tops—about 2 inches wide.
Place all the patties on a sheet of aluminum foil.
Heat 2 tablespoons butter and 2 tablespoons of oil in a large sauté pan over medium heat.
Add the keftedes and cook for 5 minutes on each side.

To make the brown butter: Melt a stick of butter over medium heat until it just turns brown.
Turn off the heat and pour over the spaghetti.

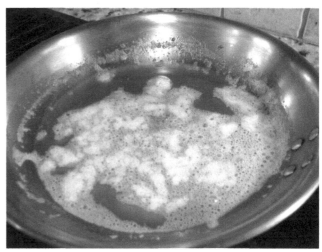

brown butter

113

NEW ORLEANS ANDOUILLE PAPPARDELLE

This is a one-pot meal that's loaded with flavor. If you don't like your food too spicy you can leave out the cayenne pepper—andouille sausage is spicy on its own. If you really want to cut down on the spice, add ½ cup cream or ½ cup sour cream to the sauce in the last 2 minutes of cooking.

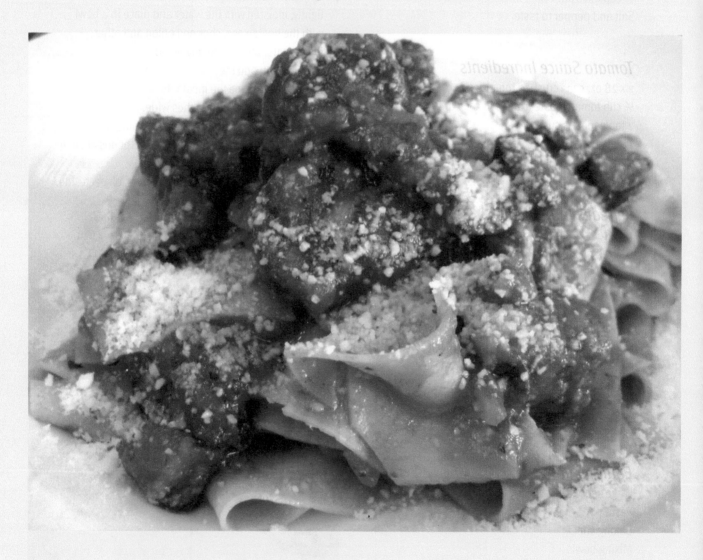

Servings: 6 - 8
Prep time: 10 minutes
Cooking time: 30 minutes
Cost: $18.44

Ingredients

1 lb. of Andouille sausage, cubed
1 yellow onion, chopped
8 oz. button mushrooms, sliced
29 oz. can of plain tomato sauce
½ cup Parmesan cheese
2 tablespoons olive oil + 2 tablespoons
2 tablespoons garlic paste
1 tablespoon dried oregano
1 teaspoon salt
¼ teaspoon cayenne pepper
½ pound pappardelle pasta (wide noodles)

Equipment

Large sauté pan
Cutting board
Measuring cups & spoons
Pasta/stock pot
Paring knife
Spatula

Directions

1. Cut the sausage into rounds, then quarter each round.
   Heat a large sauté pan over medium-high heat.
   Once the pan is hot add the oil
   Add the sausage and cook for 8-10 minutes.
   Remove the sausage and add the other 2 tablespoons
   of olive oil, onions, mushrooms, cayenne pepper,
   oregano, garlic paste, salt and cayenne pepper.

2. Reduce the heat to medium and cook for about
   10 minutes.
   When the vegetables are soft, add the tomato sauce
   and sausage and cook over medium-low heat for about
   20 minutes.

3. Cook the pasta according the package directions.
   Remember to salt the pasta water with 1-2 tablespoons
   of salt once it comes to a boil.
   Drain the pasta, add the pasta to the pan with the sauce,
   add ½ cup Parmesan cheese and serve.

MOROCCAN STUFFED SHELLS WITH CURRIED BÉCHAMEL

Moroccan flavors again? Yes! Raisins, carrots, curry, cinnamon—mixed with a creamy sauce, pasta, and cheese—yum!

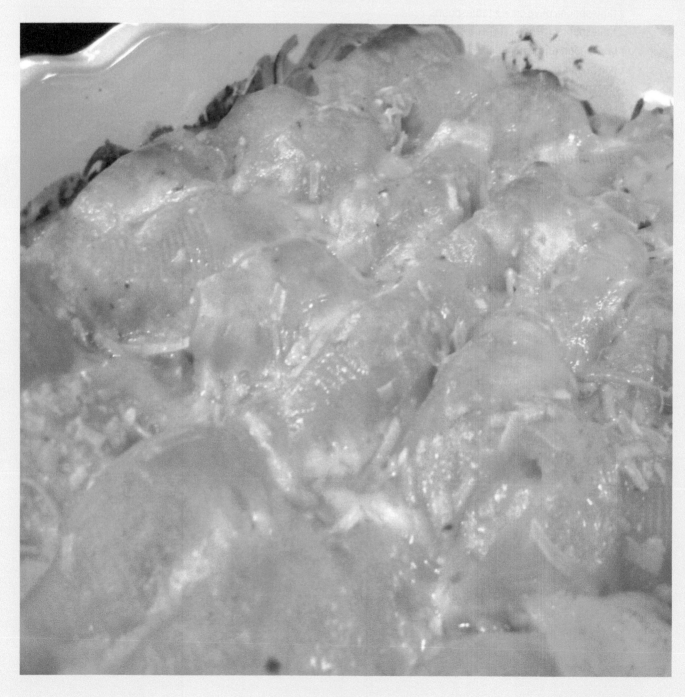

Servings: 6 - 8
Prep time: 20 minutes
Cooking time: 40 minutes
Cost: $10.84

Ingredients

24 jumbo pasta shells (8-10 ounce package)
2 cups ricotta cheese
1 cup shredded carrots
1/2 cup raisins
2 eggs
½ cup Parmesan cheese
½ teaspoon ground cinnamon
½ teaspoon salt
¼ teaspoon pepper
1 cup shredded mozzarella (for topping)
½ cup Parmesan cheese (for topping)
Béchamel sauce
4 cups milk *
4 tablespoons unsalted butter
4 tablespoons flour
1 tablespoon curry powder
1 teaspoon salt
½ teaspoon pepper

Equipment

Pasta pot
Small and large saucepans
Large mixing bowl
9x12 baking dish
Medium saucepan if you are heating your milk

Directions

1. Preheat the oven to 350 degrees F.

2. Cook shells according to package directions. After draining, let cool while you prepare the filling and sauce.

3. In a small saucepan add the carrots and 1 cup of water. Cook over medium heat for 5 minutes, drain and set aside.

4. To prepare the filling: in a large mixing bowl mix together the ricotta, carrots, raisins, egg, Parmesan, cinnamon, salt, and pepper.
   Put 1 heaping tablespoon of filling into each shell.

5. To prepare the béchamel sauce: melt the butter in a large saucepan over medium-low heat then add the flour and whisk until you have made a blond roux—this will take about 1-2 minutes.
   Add the curry and whisk for another minute.
   Slowly add the milk, whisking continuously, and raise the heat to medium-high until the sauce begins to boil—then reduce the heat to low and cook for 8-10 minutes until the sauce is thickened.

6. Pour about ½ cup of the béchamel sauce on the bottom of your baking dish then place the filled shells in the baking dish and cover with the remaining sauce.
   Sprinkle with mozzarella and Parmesan and bake for 20-25 minutes until golden on top.

   When making a béchamel sauce, some experts recommend warming the milk before adding it to the roux to prevent lumps. We've experimented using cold and warm milk and found that they both work.

ARTICHOKE PESTO ALFREDO

We've created a mellow yet rich pesto by combining a classic recipe with artichokes and cream. Toss this sauce with any of your favorite pasta shapes.

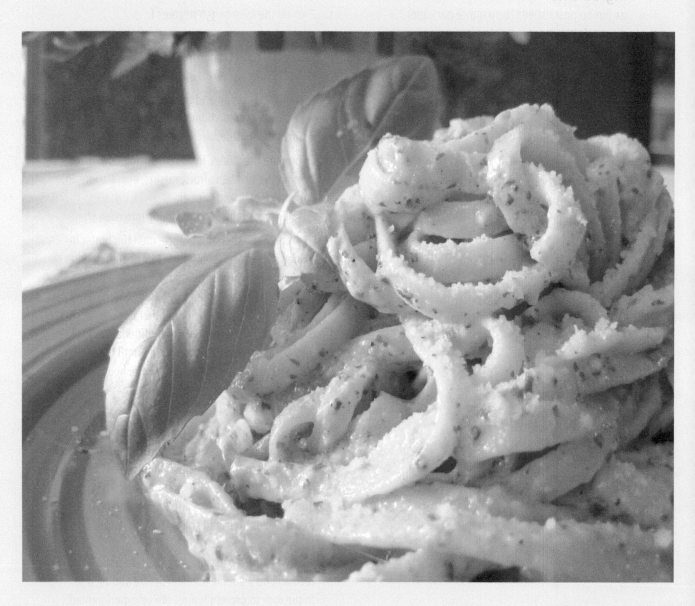

Servings: 6 - 8
Prep time: 10 minutes
Cooking time: 20 minutes
Cost: $14.52

Ingredients

1 lb. fettuccine pasta
Alfredo sauce (see below)
Pesto (see below)

Alfredo Sauce Ingredients

1 cup heavy cream
4 tablespoons unsalted butter
½ cup grated Parmesan
¼ teaspoon nutmeg
½ teaspoon pepper

Pesto Ingredients

2 cups basil leaves
4 tablespoons pine nuts
½ cup olive oil
½ cup grated Parmesan
½ teaspoon of pepper
2 teaspoons garlic paste
4 artichoke hearts

Equipment

Pasta Pot
Food processor
Medium saucepan (for the Alfredo sauce)
Whisk
Wooden spoon

Directions

1. Boil the pasta in a large boiling pot.
   While the pasta is boiling, blend the pesto
   ingredients in a food processor.
   Set the pesto aside.
   Drain the water from the pasta and set aside.

2. In a medium saucepan, heat the butter and
   heavy cream over medium-low heat and
   continue to cook until thickened, about
   6 - 8 minutes.
   Whisk thoroughly while adding the nutmeg
   and pepper.
   When the sauce has begun to thicken
   and bubble, remove it from the heat and
   add the Parmesan.
   Mix with a whisk until fully blended and
   sufficiently thick to coat the back of a wooden
   spoon.

3. Add the Alfredo sauce to the pasta and mix,
   preferably with tongs.
   Next, add the pesto sauce and mix until
   the pasta is coated with sauce.
   Serve with a sprinkle of freshly grated
   Parmesan to garnish.

CHEESE TORTELLINI WITH PUMPKIN AND FRIED SAGE

Ring in the fall season with this elegant pasta dish.
Sage has a wonderful earthy flavor that smells and tastes like Thanksgiving.

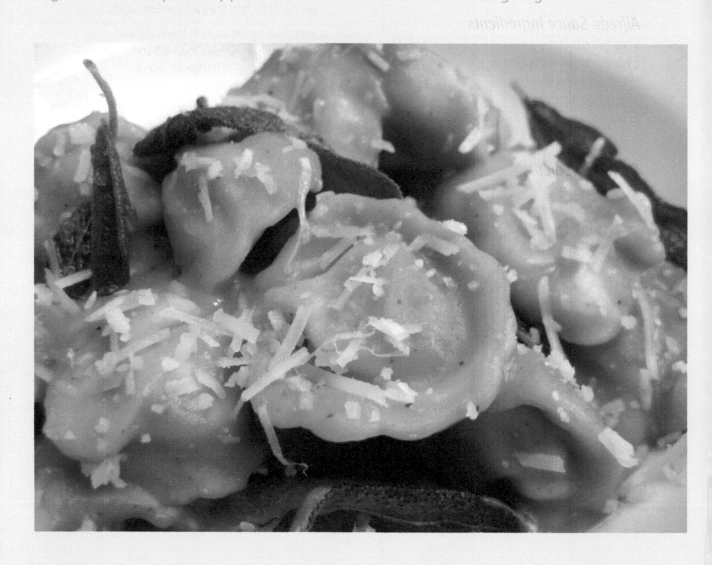

Servings: 6 - 8
Prep time: 5 minutes
Cooking time: 15 minutes
Cost: $12.95

Ingredients
16-18 oz. of prepared cheese-filled tortellini
Fried sage (see below)
Pumpkin sauce (see below)

Pumpkin Sauce
Fried Sage
1 x 15 ounce can of pumpkin
10-12 leaves of fresh sage
1 cup heavy cream or half and half
3 tablespoons olive oil
½ cup brown sugar
½ teaspoon salt
¼ teaspoon black pepper
¼ teaspoon nutmeg (optional)
¼ teaspoon ground cinnamon

Equipment
Pasta pot
Medium saucepan (for the pumpkin sauce)
Small saucepan or small sauté pan (for the fried sage)

Directions
1. Mix the pumpkin sauce ingredients together in a saucepan over medium-low heat for 10 minutes.

2. In a small sauté pan, heat 3 tablespoons of olive oil over medium heat and add the sage leaves and cook for 1-2 minutes. * Butter would also work well here.

3. Cook the tortellini according to package directions. Drain the pasta then cover with sauce and sage leaves.

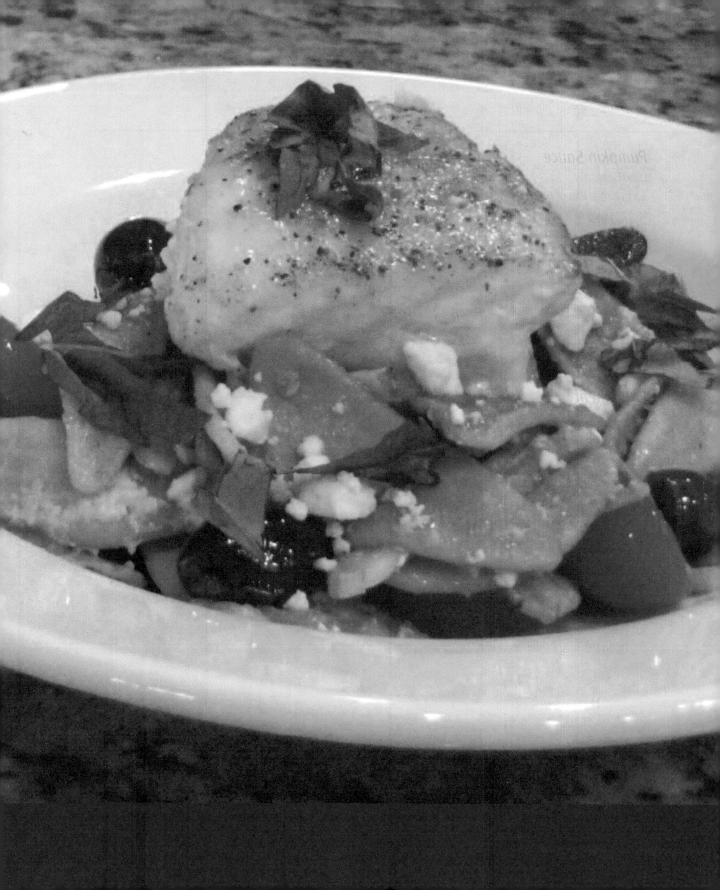

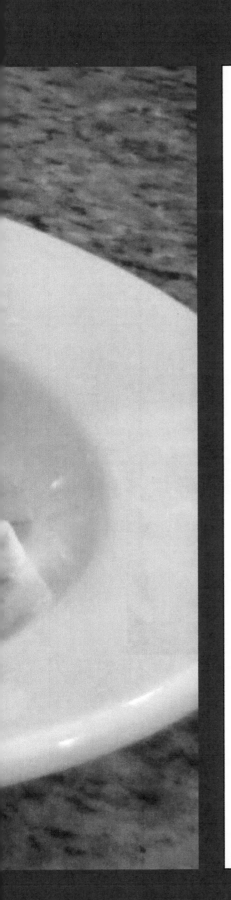

Garlic Shrimp Orzo

Choco-chili

Salmon Risotto with Caper Cream Sauce

Filet Mignon with Truffled Mashed Potatoes

21st Century Pork Chops and Apple Sauce

*Yia-Yia's Chicken Tenders with Homemade Honey
    Mustard Sauce*

New Orleans Shrimp Étouffée

Seared Tuna Tacos

*Coconut Pecan Crusted Tilapia with Warm Mango
    Pineapple Salsa*

Seared Bass on Artisanal Pasta

Angel Citrus Salmon

GARLIC SHRIMP ORZO

This addictive and quick dish can dress up any dinner or lunch date.

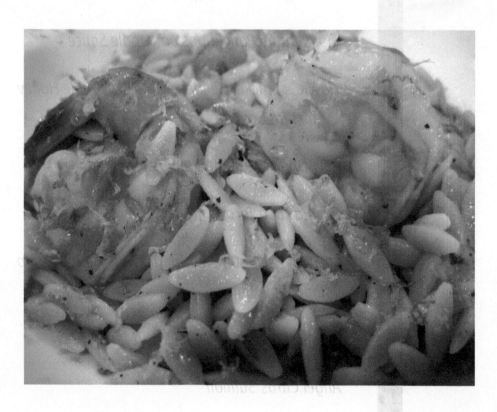

Servings: 4
Prep time: 15 minutes
Cooking time: 15 minutes
Cost: $15.33

Ingredients

1 lb. de-shelled, de-veined shrimp
3 cups orzo (this is pasta; it's in the pasta aisle)
6 – 8 cloves of garlic, finely chopped
2 tablespoons + 3 tablespoons of olive oil
2 tablespoons of butter
Zest of 1 lemon and 1 lime
¼ cup lemon juice (juice of 1 fresh lemon)
¼ cup lime juice (juice of 1 fresh lime)
1 teaspoon salt + 1 teaspoon salt
½ teaspoon black pepper

Equipment

Pasta pot
Large sauté pan
Microplane/"Zester"
Large wooden spoon
Chopping or paring knife
Cutting board

Directions

1. Cook the orzo as per directions on the package.
   Remember to salt the water once it has come to a boil;
   this is your only chance to season pasta.
   After draining, add 3 tablespoons of olive oil and
   1 teaspoon of salt.
   Allow it to sit with heat off while preparing the shrimp.
   Cover the pot with a lid or foil to keep it warm.

2. Chop 6 – 8 cloves of garlic finely. Preheat a large sauté
   pan over medium-high heat. Once the pan is hot, add
   the garlic, 2 tablespoons of butter, and 2 tablespoons
   of olive oil and sauté.
   Do not allow the garlic to cook for more than 30 seconds.
   Burnt garlic is very bitter.

3. Add in the shrimp, lemon juice, lime juice, zest, 1 teaspoon
   salt, and pepper to the pan and cook for 4 – 5 minutes
   (if you are using the juice in a plastic container, add
   ¼ cup lemon juice and ¼ cup lime juice).
   To really enhance the citrus flavor, you can toss the
   halves of lemon and lime directly into the pan and
   sauté along with the shrimp.
   Make sure to turn the shrimp so that it cooks on
   both sides. When the shrimp turns pink it is cooked.
   Add the orzo directly to the pan with the shrimp and mix.

4. For the final touch of flavor, add and mix 1 teaspoon of
   salt and ½ teaspoon of pepper.
   Your shrimp is ready to serve!

CHOCO-CHILI

Our sweet and spicy twist on the classic.

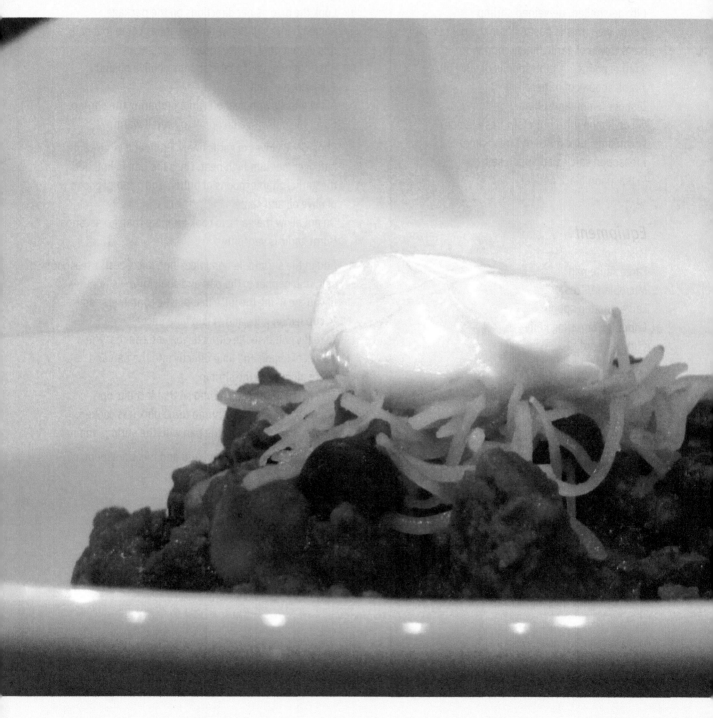

Servings: 8 – 10
Prep time: 5 minutes
Cooking time: 1 hour 30 minutes
Cost: $11.97

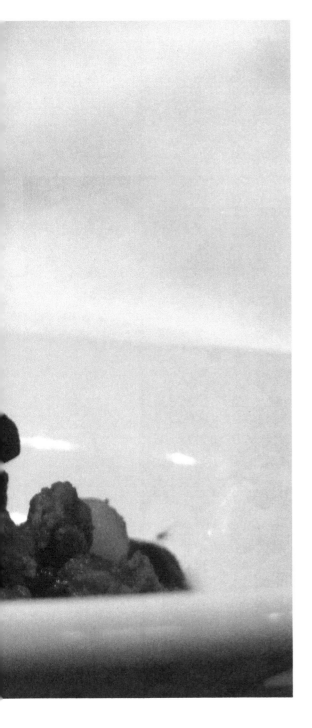

Ingredients

1 cup chocolate chips (preferably dark chocolate)
2 cans dark red kidney beans (15.5 oz. cans)
1 can garbanzo beans (15.5 oz. can)
1 can black beans (15.5 oz. can)
2 cans crushed tomatoes (28 oz. can)
2 lbs ground beef (cheapest is $1.99 a pound)
½ teaspoon cayenne pepper
1 teaspoon salt x 2
½ teaspoon black pepper x 2
2 tablespoons of vegetable oil
Shredded cheddar or Monterey jack for garnish
Sour cream for garnish

Equipment

Large stock pot or pasta pot
Can opener
Wooden spoon
Measuring spoons

Directions

1. Add 2 tablespoons of oil to a large stockpot.
   Add the ground beef and brown over medium-low heat
   until cooked, about 15 minutes.

2. While cooking, break the meat into small pieces with
   a spatula or large cooking spoon. Season the meat with
   1 teaspoon of salt, ½ teaspoon of cayenne, and ½
   teaspoon of black pepper.

3. Once the meat is cooked, add the cans of beans and
   crushed tomato. Be sure to drain the juice from the
   bean cans; otherwise, you'll have a very soupy chili.

4. Season the mixture with another 1 teaspoon of salt
   and ½ teaspoon of black pepper.

5. Lower heat to medium-low and cook for 30 – 45 minutes.
   Just before serving, add 1 cup of chocolate chips and
   stir until melted.
   Serve in a bowl and garnish with shredded cheese
   and sour cream as desired.

Salmon Risotto With Caper Cream Sauce

Don't let anyone tell you a beginner cook can't make risotto!!
If you follow our easy steps, you won't only be able to make this recipe;
you will also be able to substitute a multitude of ingredients for many,
many interesting risotto dishes. The only things you will need are 4 pans
and 20 minutes of your undivided time.
Not that much for an incredible meal.

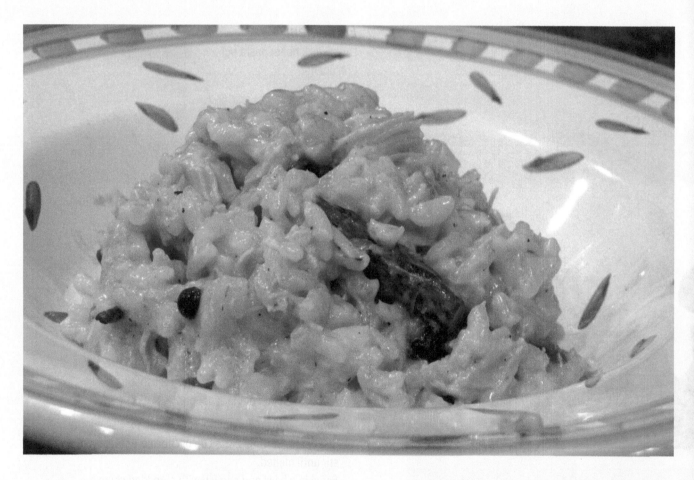

Servings: 4 - 6
Prep time: 10 minutes
Cooking time: 40 minutes
Cost: $20.21

Ingredients

½ lb. salmon, deboned and de-skinned (leftovers are great for this dish)

½ cup asparagus cut in 1 inch pieces

2 cups risotto rice (Arborio)

1 cup heavy cream

6 cups chicken or vegetable broth

1/3 cup small capers, drained

1 tablespoon unsalted butter

1 onion, chopped

4 cloves of garlic, finely chopped (use 2 table-spoons if using the paste in a tube)

¼ cup olive oil + 1 tbsp olive oil

1 teaspoon salt *

½ teaspoon black pepper

Equipment

Large and medium sized sauté pans (for the risotto, salmon, and asparagus)

1 ½ to 2 quart sauce pan (for the cream sauce)

4 or more quart sauce pan (for the chicken broth)

Measuring cups and spoons

Soup ladle and large stirring spoons

Directions

To make the asparagus:

Sauté the asparagus with 1 tablespoon oil over medium heat for 5 minutes. Only use the top half of the asparagus stem—the bottom half is very tough.

Turn off the heat and set aside in a bowl.

You can use this same pan for cooking the salmon.

To make the salmon:

Heat the asparagus pan over medium heat.

Once the pan is hot, add the salmon and cook for 2 minutes. Flip the salmon, cover, and turn down the heat to medium-low. Cook for 8-10 minutes. Then cut into cubes and set aside.

To make the cream sauce: Heat a saucepan over medium heat and add the butter, garlic, and capers and cook for 2 minutes. Next add the cream and bring to a boil over medium-high heat. When the sauce comes to a boil, turn down the heat to low and cook for 10 minutes, stirring occasionally. The sauce will be ready when it is thick enough to coat the back of a spoon.

To make the risotto:

Heat the chicken broth in a large saucepan over medium heat for 5 minutes. Meanwhile, sauté the chopped onions in ¼ cup olive oil over medium heat for 5-8 minutes until they are soft and translucent. Add the risotto rice to the pan with the onions and stir for 2 minutes. Then begin adding the chicken broth—use a soup ladle for this.

Add enough to just cover the rice, stir continuously until the broth is absorbed. Then add more, and repeat this process until all the broth has been used.

It will take about 18-20 minutes.

Once the risotto is done, add the pepper, asparagus, salmon, and cream sauce. Stir and serve.

* Wait until the entire dish is complete before seasoning.

The chicken broth and capers both have salt.

You will likely not need any extra salt.

For basic risotto:

Use a 3:1 ratio of broth to rice. Sauté onions or shallots and ¼ cup olive oil in large sauté pan over medium heat for 5 to 8 minutes. Add the rice and cook for 2-3 minutes until the rice is coated with the olive oil.

Add the broth in batches—enough each time to cover the rice—once the broth is absorbed, add more until it is all used. Done!! Serve like this or add sautéed mushrooms and Parmesan, or sautéed pancetta and artichoke hearts, etc., etc.

FILET MIGNON WITH TRUFFLED MASHED POTATOES

Restaurant quality elegance and taste at home. Use any cut of meat you like here. If you want to splurge for a fresh black truffle (will run you about $20-25), use your grater to grate fresh truffle over your meat and potatoes.

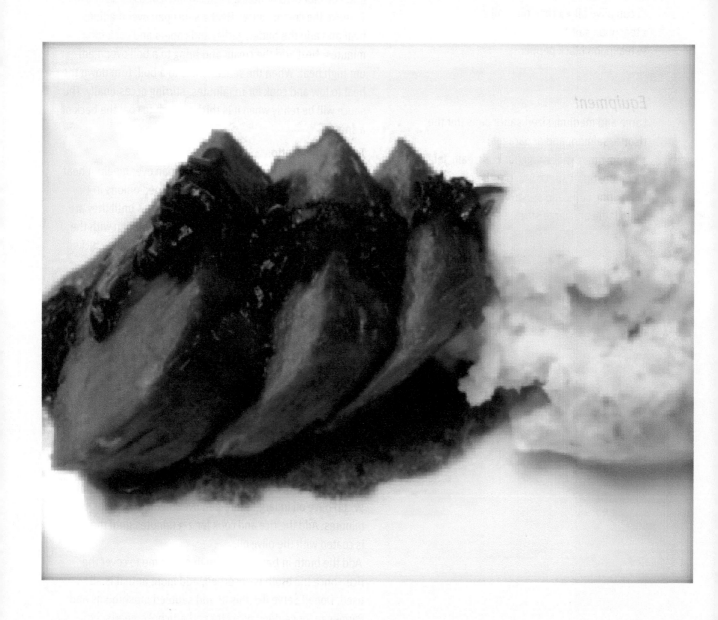

Servings: 4
Prep time: 15 minutes
Cooking time: 20 minutes
Cost: $19.65

Ingredients

1 lb. filet mignon or NY strip steak
2 tablespoons olive oil
Truffled mashed potatoes (see below)
Balsamic reduction (see below)

Truffled Mashed Potatoes

4 Yukon Gold potatoes, peeled and cubed
½ cup cream or half and half
4 tablespoons unsalted butter
1 tablespoon truffle oil
1 teaspoon salt (+extra for seasoning meat)
½ teaspoon pepper (+extra for seasoning meat)

Balsamic Reduction Sauce
½ cup balsamic vinegar
2 shallots
2 teaspoons sugar
1 teaspoon butter

Equipment

Medium sauté pan, with oven-safe handles
Small saucepan, for reduction
Large saucepan or pasta pot, for potatoes

Directions

Preheat the oven to 400 degrees F.

For the meat:
Heat a medium size sauté pan over medium heat.
Once the pan is hot add the olive oil. Sprinkle the meat on each side with salt and pepper.
Sear the meat for 1 minute on each side.
Turn off the heat and place the pan in the oven: cook 8 minutes for medium rare, 10 minutes for medium, 12 minutes for medium well.
Remove from the oven and slice pieces into 1-inch pieces.

For the balsamic reduction:
Put all ingredients in a small saucepan and bring to a boil over medium-high heat. Once it begins to boil, reduce the heat to medium-low and cook until thick---about 8-10 minutes.

To cook the potatoes:
Place potatoes in a saucepan in cold water (use enough water to cover the potatoes).
Bring to a boil and cook until the potatoes are fork-tender—about 15 minutes.
Drain, place in a mixing bowl and add cream, butter, truffle oil, salt and pepper and mash with a potato masher until smooth.

To plate:
Slice the meat in 1 inch thick slices, drizzle with balsamic reduction. Serve alongside mashed potatoes.

21St Century Pork Chops and Apple Sauce

We've taken this classic 60's meal and updated it with pomegranate sautéed apples and roasted blue potatoes. And you can have it on the table in 30 minutes.

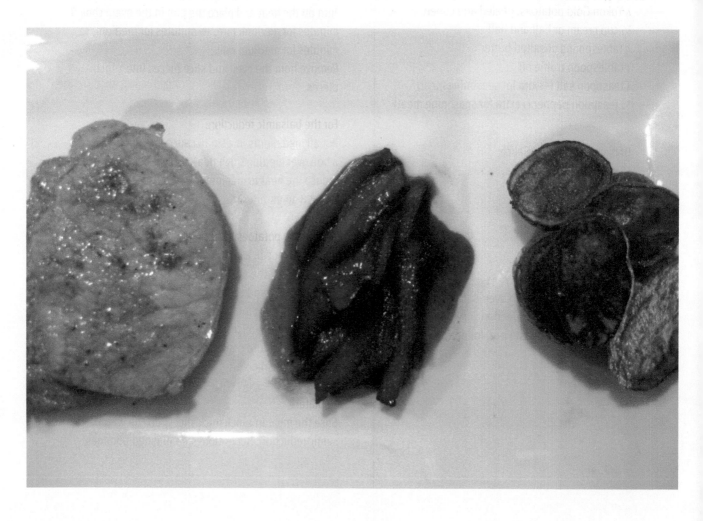

Servings: 4
Prep time: 20 minutes
Cooking time: 25 minutes
Cost: $16.16

Ingredients

Pork
1 pound of boneless, thin cut pork chops
Pork marinade:
½ cup rice wine vinegar
½ cup oil (olive or vegetable)
2 tablespoons Worcestershire sauce
1 teaspoon salt
½ teaspoon black pepper
½ teaspoon garlic powder
½ teaspoon onion powder
½ teaspoon Chinese five spice

Apples
3 apples
1 cup pomegranate juice
1 tablespoon butter
1 tablespoon lemon juice

Potatoes
1 ½ pound bag of baby purple potatoes
2 tablespoons olive oil
2 teaspoons salt
1 teaspoon black pepper

Equipment

Medium sauté pan
Broiler pan
Baking pan
Mixing bowls
Measuring spoons & cups
Chopping/paring knife

Directions

Preheat the oven to 400 degrees F.

For the pork chops: mix the marinade ingredients together in a mixing bowl and add the pork.
Place in the refrigerator for 15 to 20 minutes.

For the potatoes: wash and cut the blue potatoes in half and place on a baking sheet. Drizzle with oil, salt, and pepper and bake at 400 degrees for 20 to 25 minutes until golden brown. After the potatoes have been taken out of the oven, set the oven to broil.

For the apples: peel and thinly slice the apples, place in a bowl and cover with lemon juice.
Heat the butter in a sauté pan over medium heat. Add the apples and the pomegranate juice and cook for about 15 minutes until the apples are tender and the juice has thickened.

Place the pork on a broiler pan and broil for 2 minutes per side. Add more marinade when you turn the meat.
Do not serve this marinade with the cooked meat — it had the raw pork in it!

YIA-YIA'S CHICKEN TENDERS WITH HOMEMADE HONEY MUSTARD SAUCE

Warm or cold, you won't be able to get enough of these. Plain, on a sandwich, in a salad, at 3 pm or 3 am, these will be an instant favorite. The honey mustard also goes great on salads and fresh veggies.

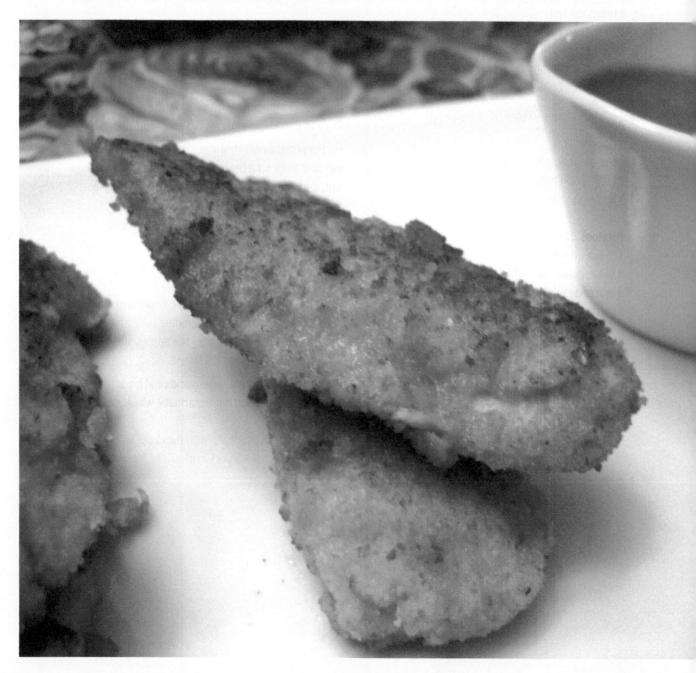

Servings: 4
Prep time: 10 minutes
Cooking time: 10 minutes
Cost: $10.18

Ingredients

1 ½ pounds chicken tenders
2 large eggs, beaten
2 cups bread crumbs
2 tablespoons unsalted butter
2 tablespoons olive oil
Juice of 1 lemon (for marinating chicken)

Honey Mustard Sauce Ingredients

½ cup Dijon mustard
10 tablespoons honey
4 tablespoons ketchup
2 tablespoons pomegranate juice
½ teaspoon salt
¼ teaspoon pepper

Equipment

Large sauté pan
Small mixing bowl for honey mustard
2 large bowls—1 for eggs and 1 for breadcrumbs
Measuring cups & spoons

Directions

1. Place the eggs in one of the large bowls and the breadcrumbs in the other. Set them next to the stove to make for easy breading of the chicken.

2. Rinse the raw chicken under cold water. Be sure to remove the tendons from the raw meat. Squeeze the juice of 1 lemon over the chicken. Ideally you want to let the lemon tenderize the meat for 20-30 minutes.

3. Heat a large sauté pan over medium heat with the olive oil and butter. Dip the chicken first in the egg, then in the breadcrumbs. Lay the strips onto the pan until browned, about 4 – 5 minutes on each side.

4. To make the mustard sauce: Whisk all ingredients in a bowl and use for dipping.

NEW ORLEANS SHRIMP ÉTOUFFÉE

This is a classic New Orleans dish. Étouffée in French means, "smothered." In this case the rice is smothered with the shrimp and sauce. It's similar to gumbo, but thicker; it is usually made with seafood such as crab or crawfish, but can be made with meats as well.

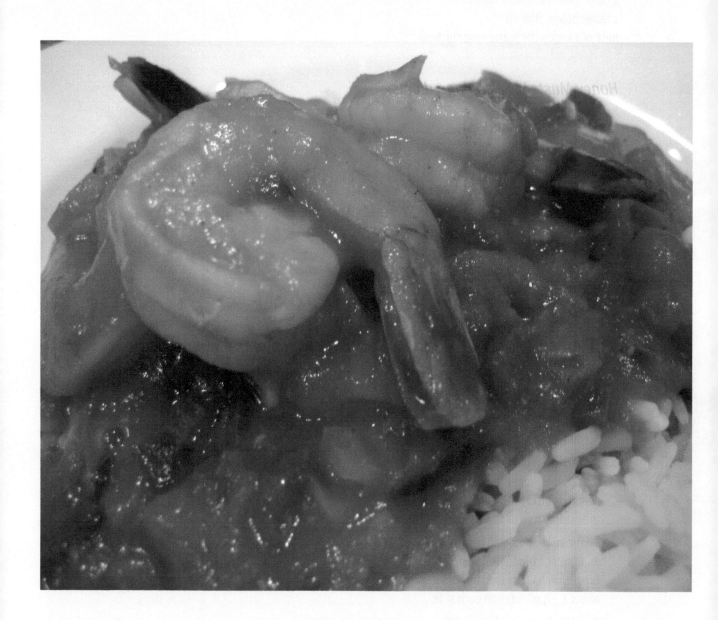

Servings: 6 - 8
Prep time: 15 minutes
Cooking time: 1 hour
Cost: $27.86

Ingredients
2 pounds 21-25 raw, deveined shrimp (21-25 shrimp per lb.—medium-sized)
1 stick unsalted butter
4 tablespoons flour
1 yellow onion, diced
1 green pepper, diced
2 stalks large, or 4 stalks small celery stalks, diced
2 x 28 oz. cans of diced tomatoes
1 cup water
2 tablespoons garlic paste (or 4 cloves)
2 teaspoons salt
1 teaspoon black pepper
¼ teaspoon cayenne pepper
Long grain rice (follow package directions for number of guests)

Equipment
Large stockpot
Medium saucepan for the rice
Can opener
Wooden spoon

Directions
1. In a medium saucepan cook the rice according to how many guests you have. This recipe will easily serve as a main course.

2. Melt the butter in a large stockpot over medium heat, add the flour, and cook until you have made a dark blonde roux (the mixture will look light brown)—this takes about 4-5 minutes.

3. Add the onion, celery, and pepper (referred to as "the trinity" in New Orleans cuisine), and cook for 10 minutes. Add the tomatoes and water and cook over medium-low heat for 30 minutes to allow all the flavors to marry and for the sauce to thicken.

4. Once the sauce is thick, turn up the heat to medium, add the shrimp and cook for another 7-8 minutes.

5. Serve in bowls. Put the rice down first then spoon étouffée generously over the rice.

SEARED TUNA TACOS

Tuna in a taco? Yes indeed. A modern day twist on the soft taco. Light, healthy, and low-cal.

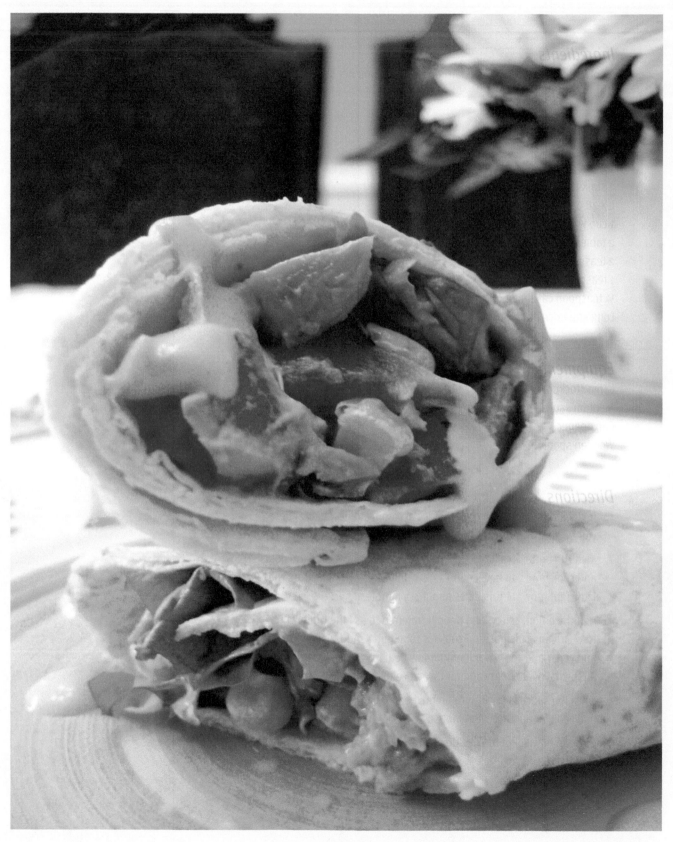

Servings: 4
Prep time: 10 minutes
Cooking time: 3 minutes
Cost: $27.91

Ingredients

1 lb fresh sashimi grade tuna (ask fishmonger)
2 cups lettuce, chopped
2 avocados, cubed or diced
4 soft taco shells
2 tablespoons olive oil
1 cup canned corn
Sauce (see below)

Sauce Ingredients

2 heaping tablespoons mayonnaise
1 tablespoon lemon juice
½ teaspoon wasabi paste
1 teaspoon sesame oil
2 teaspoons soy sauce

Equipment

Large sauté pan
Mixing bowl
Measuring cups & spoons

Directions

1. Heat an empty, large sauté pan over medium-low heat. Heat each taco shell for one minute on each side.
   If you want to have the shells heated when the tuna is ready, use another pan to sear the tuna.
   If not, the same pan will do.

2. In a mixing bowl, combine the sauce ingredients and stir until it reaches a smooth, sauce-like consistency and is thoroughly blended.
   Dice the avocados and chop the lettuce.

3. For searing the tuna: Heat 2 tablespoons olive oil in a large sauté pan over medium-high heat.
   Season the tuna with salt and pepper on each side.
   Sear for about 90 seconds on each side.
   Dice the tuna once it is cooked.
   The less time you sear, the less cooked your tuna will be, and vice-versa.
   If you ask your local fishmonger for true sashimi grade tuna, you should not worry about parasites or disease.
   If it is not sashimi grade, we recommend cooking the tuna the entire way through.

4. To build your taco: fill the warm tortilla shells with the avocado, tuna, corn, lettuce, and dressing, wrap, and serve!

Coconut Pecan Crusted Tilapia With Warm Mango Pineapple Salsa

Tilapia is an inexpensive, readily available fish. It's very light and bland in flavor and therefore requires some bold accompaniments. We've given it a Hawaiian flavor with coconut and pineapple.

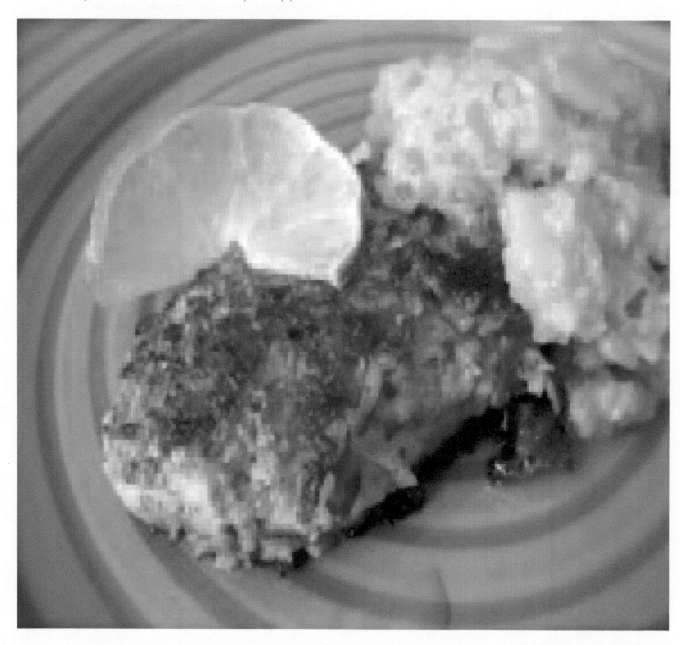

Servings: 4
Prep time: 15 minutes
Cooking time: 10 minutes
Cost: $12.20

Pecan Coating Ingredients

½ cup pecan nuts, chopped in a food processor *
¼ cup bread crumbs
½ cup coconut milk
½ cup shredded coconut

Fish Ingredients

2 tablespoons unsalted butter
2 tablespoons olive oil
1 lb. fresh tilapia, cut into 4 pieces

Tropical Salsa Ingredients

1 teaspoon lime juice (fresh or bottled)
½ cup pineapple chunks (sweetened—comes in 8 oz. cans)
1 ripe mango, peeled and cubed
¼ cup cilantro, chopped
Pinch of salt
Pinch of pepper

Equipment

Large sauté pan
Small saucepan
Paring knife
Mixing bowls for coating the fish (pie plates work great here)
Measuring cups & spoons
Food processor

Directions

1. Heat a large sauté pan over medium-high heat with the butter and olive oil.

2. Set aside 2 separate bowls: mix the chopped pecan nuts, shredded coconut, and breadcrumbs in one, and add coconut milk to the other.
    Salt and pepper the fish on each side.
    Dunk the fish first in the coconut milk, then into the pecan coating.
    Sear in the pan for 5 minutes per side over medium-high.

3. Blend the salsa ingredients in a food processor until the consistency is chunky.
    If you are not using a food processor you can cut the fruit into small cubes and mix the salsa ingredients with a spoon.
    In a small saucepan, heat over medium-low heat for about 5 minutes, stirring occasionally.

* If you don't have a food processor you can put the nuts in a zip lock baggie and crush them with a rolling pin or a big book.

To serve: plate the fish and top with the warm salsa.

SEARED BASS ON ARTISANAL PASTA

Don't be scared by the cost on this one—if you ordered this dish in a restaurant it would be $28 per person! We recommend artisanal pasta to dress up the flavors and colors. Artisan means craftsman, and the word artisanal refers to the art of making something by hand. This is why artisanal products are usually more expensive than mass-produced products.

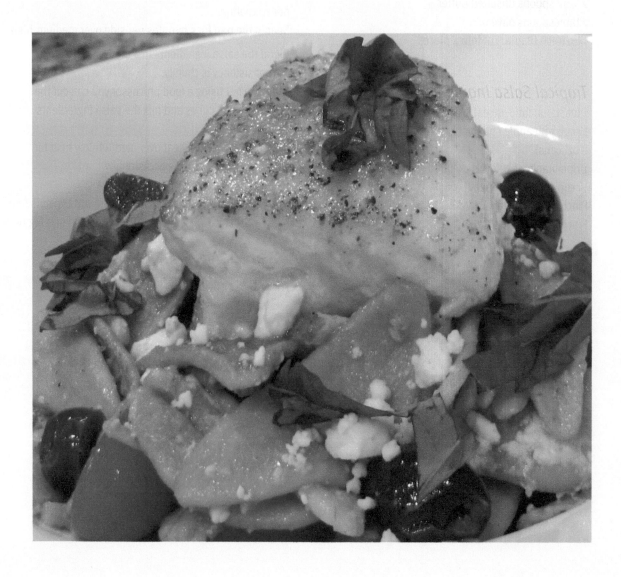

Servings: 4
Prep time: 20 minutes
Cooking time: 35 minutes
Cost: $36.13

Ingredients

1 pound bass fish, cut into 4 pieces
1 pound artisanal tricolor pasta
1 cup black olives (preferably Kalamata),
    rough chop
1 cup grape tomatoes (sliced in half)
1 cup crumbled feta cheese
1 large fennel bulb, sliced thinly
2 shallots, finely chopped
3 cloves garlic, finely chopped
    (or 1 ½ tablespoons garlic paste)
¼ cup olive oil + 2 tablespoons + 3 tablespoons
2 tablespoons balsamic vinegar
2 tablespoons fresh basil for garnish (optional)
½ teaspoon salt (+ pinch for seasoning fish)
¼ teaspoon pepper (+ pinch for seasoning fish)

Equipment

Pasta Pot
2 sauté pans (1 large & 1 medium)
Measuring cups & spoons
Paring knife
Spatula

Directions

1. Preheat the oven to 375 degrees F.

2. To make the fennel sauce, in a large sauté pan, sauté the fennel with ¼ cup olive oil over medium-low heat for 10 minutes, then add the shallots, garlic, salt, and pepper and cook for 5 minutes.

3. Heat a medium sauté pan over medium heat. Once the pan is hot (about 2 minutes), add the olive oil. Once the oil is hot add the fish (you will know the oil is hot when it begins to shimmer). Sear for 2 to 3 minutes per side then place in the oven for 10 minutes.
Secret tip: remember that you will not properly sear the fish if the pan and oil are not hot.

4. Cook the pasta according to the package directions. Generously salt the pasta water as it is coming to a boil (2-3 tablespoons of Kosher salt).

5. Once the pasta is done, drain and add it to the pan with the fennel.
Add 3 tablespoons olive oil and 2 tablespoons balsamic vinegar and mix well.
Next add the feta, olives, and tomatoes and turn off the heat.

6. To serve, plate each dish with a 4-ounce bass filet on top of pasta and finish with fresh basil. Drizzle each plate with olive oil.

Angel Citrus Salmon

An Asian inspired salmon dish. Low-cal, simple, and elegant. You can substitute shrimp or chicken for an equally light and delicious meal. You'll feel like you're in a restaurant on Jackson Street in San Francisco's Chinatown.

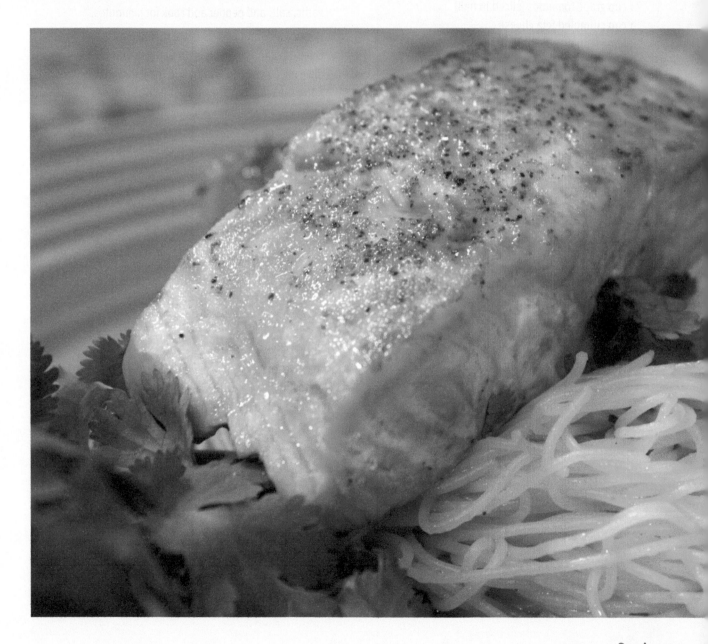

Servings: 4
Prep time: 10 minutes
Cooking time: 20 minutes
Cost: $13.19

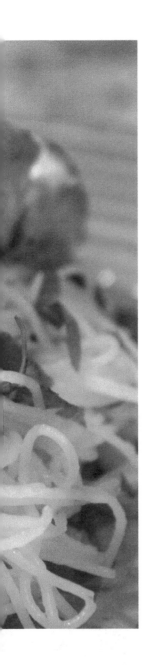

Salmon Ingredients
1 lb. salmon, cut into 4 pieces
2 tablespoons olive oil

Pasta and Pasta Sauce Ingredients
1 lb. angel hair pasta
1 shallot, sliced finely
3 cloves garlic, minced (or 1 ½ tablespoons garlic paste)
¼ cup olive oil
2 tablespoons unsalted butter
¼ cup fresh cilantro, chopped
¼ cup lemon juice (juice of 1 lemon)

Citrus Soy Glaze Ingredients
½ cup orange juice
Juice of 1 lemon
Juice of 1 lime
1 tablespoon soy sauce
¼ teaspoon ground black pepper

Equipment
Pasta Pot
2 small saucepans
Large sauté pan
Measuring cups & spoons

Directions
1. Boil the pasta as per package directions.

2. To make the pasta sauce: cook the shallots, olive oil,
    and butter over medium-low heat in a small saucepan.
    After 2 minutes, add the minced garlic and lemon juice.
    Sauté for about 1 minute. (The sauce may look broken
    but that's ok.)
    Once the pasta has boiled, drain and add the sauce to the
    pasta and mix with tongs. Top with fresh cilantro.

3. To make the citrus glaze: in a small saucepan, cook the citrus
    glaze ingredients over medium heat for 5 minutes until
    reduced and thickened. Set aside.

4. To cook the salmon: heat a large sauté pan over medium-high
    heat, add 2 tablespoons olive oil and cook the salmon for
    5-6 minutes on each side.

5. To plate: Place pasta on the center of a plate.
    Top with salmon. Then finish with a drizzle of citrus glaze
    over the salmon.

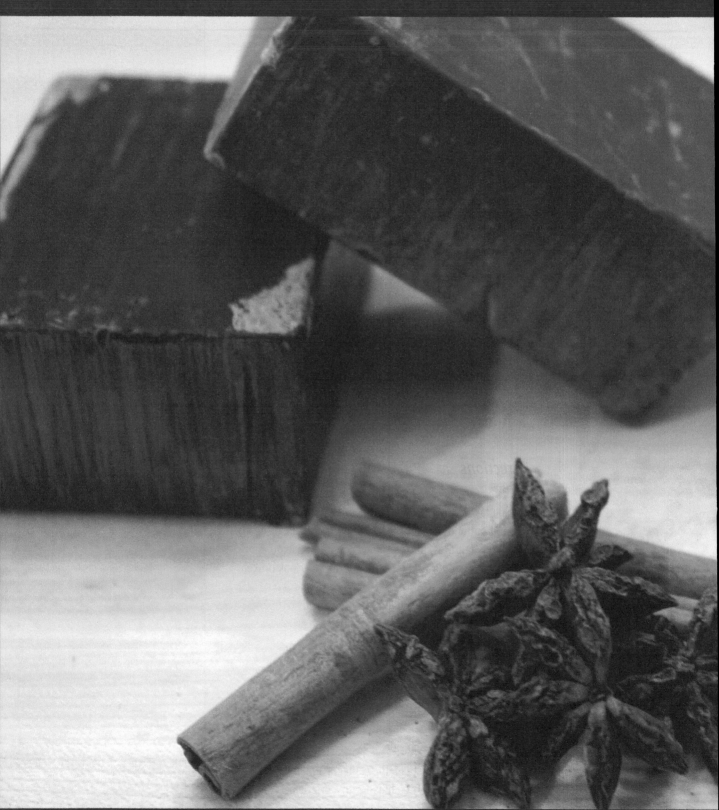

GREEK HONEY YOGURT

Yogurt for dessert? Yes! We call this our Greek "ice cream." The sugar and honey balance the tartness of the yogurt and the almond extract adds a unique cookie-like flavor to this refreshing and healthy dessert. Greek yogurt is available in most grocery stores today and can be found in the health food/organic area of your market. Perfect for a light dessert after a heavy dinner or even as a mid-day or midnight snack! It's also great for breakfast served over granola.

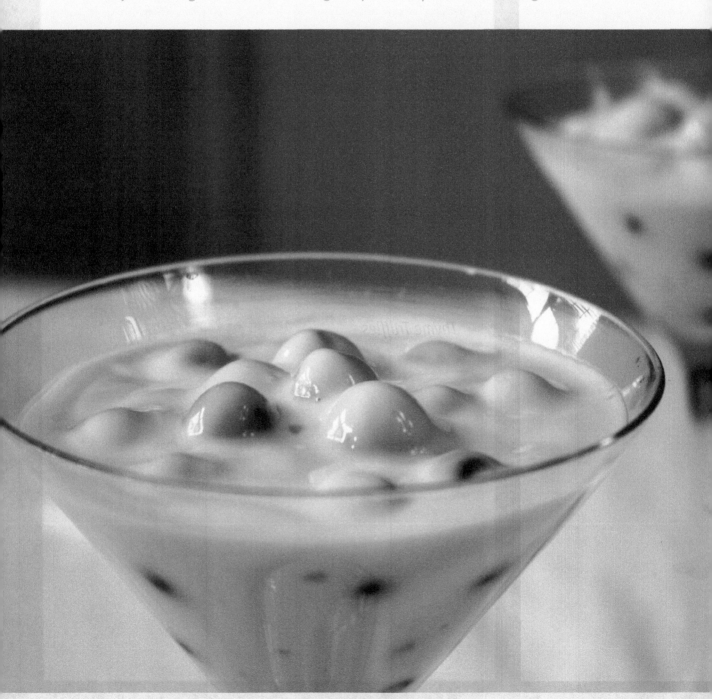

Servings: 4 – 6
Prep time: 5 minutes
Cooking time: 0 minutes
Cost: $7.98

Ingredients
2 cups plain Greek yogurt
2 cups seedless grapes
2 tablespoons honey
½ teaspoon almond extract
½ teaspoon vanilla extract
2 tablespoons superfine sugar
2 tablespoons pomegranate juice

Equipment
Mixing bowl
Spoon
Measuring cups & spoons

Directions
Always stir the yogurt while it's in its container; this helps to smooth out the texture before transferring it to another dish. In a large mixing bowl, combine all the ingredients and stir. Serve room temperature or chilled.

WHITE CHOCOLATE MACADAMIA COOKIES

More exotic refreshing Hawaiian flavors. We dress up your basic sugar cookie and make a bakery quality cookie at home. Serve this after our Coconut Crusted Tilapia and your guests will feel like they're in Maui.

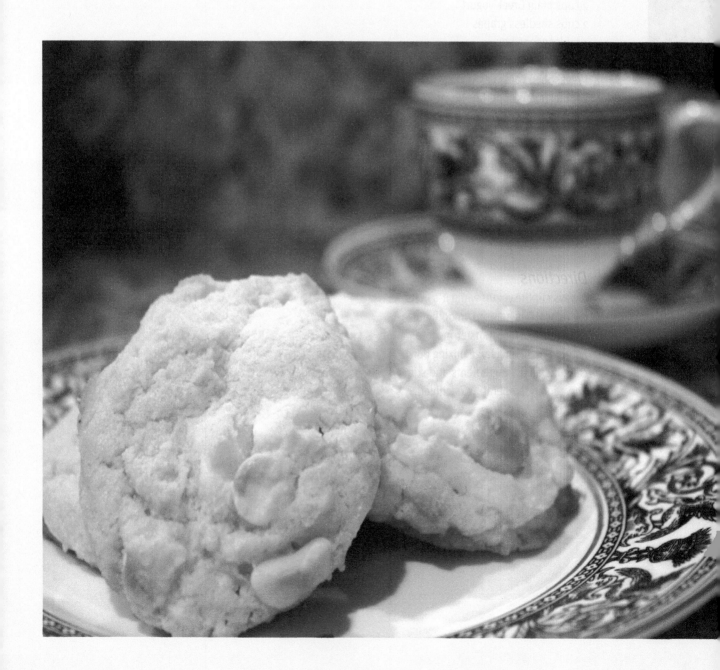

Servings: makes 14 large cookies
Prep time: 5 minutes
Cooking time: 14 minutes per batch
Cost: $8.73

Ingredients
1 x 17.5 oz. package sugar cookie mix
1 stick unsalted butter, melted
1 egg
1 teaspoon almond extract
½ cup macadamia nuts
½ cup white chocolate chips
2 tablespoons coconut milk

Equipment
Mixing bowl
Baking sheet
Parchment paper (optional, makes for easy clean-up)
Measuring cups & spoons

Directions
1. Preheat the oven to 375 degrees F.

2. Mix the coconut milk with a spoon when you first open the can.

3. Melt 1 stick of butter in a pan or in the microwave for 45 seconds. Add the melted butter and 1 egg to the cookie mix and stir until smooth.
   Add the remainder of the ingredients and mix. Form into balls on a baking sheet with parchment paper and bake for 14 minutes, until the edges become brown.

* Money saving tip: use your leftover coconut milk to make our papaya salad or our coconut pecan crusted tilapia.

For uniform cookie size use an ice cream scoop.

LEMON PUFF TARTS

These tarts are great for a spring dinner party. For a different flavor, fill these pre-made tarts with other delicious fillings like chocolate and peanut butter or fresh fruit and mascarpone cheese.

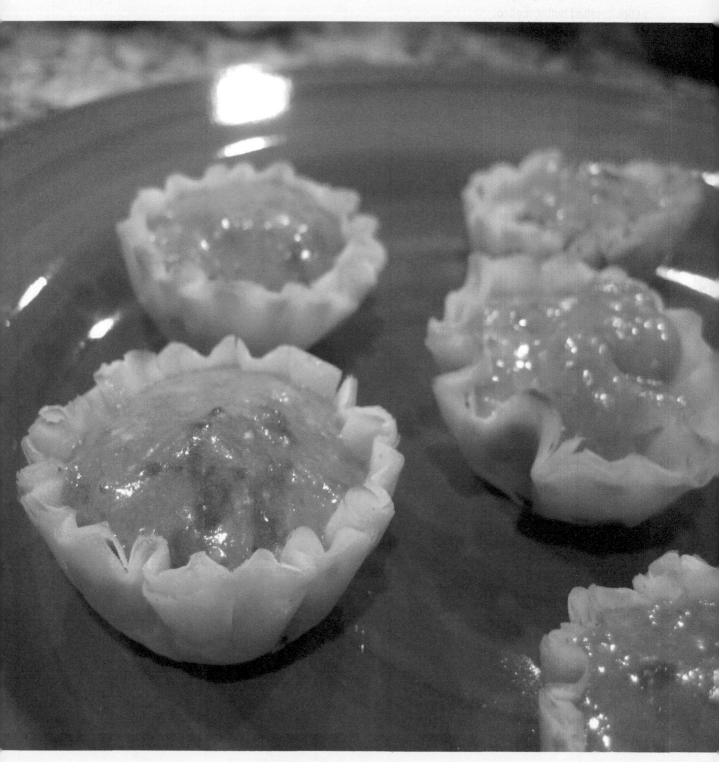

Servings: 4 - 6
Prep time: 10 minutes
Cooking time: 5 – 8 minutes
Cost: $3.45

Ingredients
1 package mini-phyllo shells (15 per pack)
¼ cup cream cheese
¼ cup blueberry preserves
2 ½ tablespoons lemon curd
    (comes jarred in jelly section of the market)

Equipment
Baking sheet
Small mixing bowl
Measuring cups & spoons
Parchment paper

Directions
1. Preheat the oven to 350 degrees F.

2. Thaw the phyllo shells according to the package directions.

3. Mix the cream cheese with blueberries in a mixing bowl and blend well.
Place ½ teaspoon lemon curd in the bottom of the shell and then place ½ teaspoon of the compound cream cheese on top of the lemon curd and bake for 6 minutes or until shells have browned (a compound cream cheese is plain cream cheese mixed with other flavors such as preserves, herbs, or vegetables). Serve warm.

MINT FUDGE BROWNIES

If you like mint you'll love these brownies. They are wonderful at holiday time sprinkled with crushed candy canes.

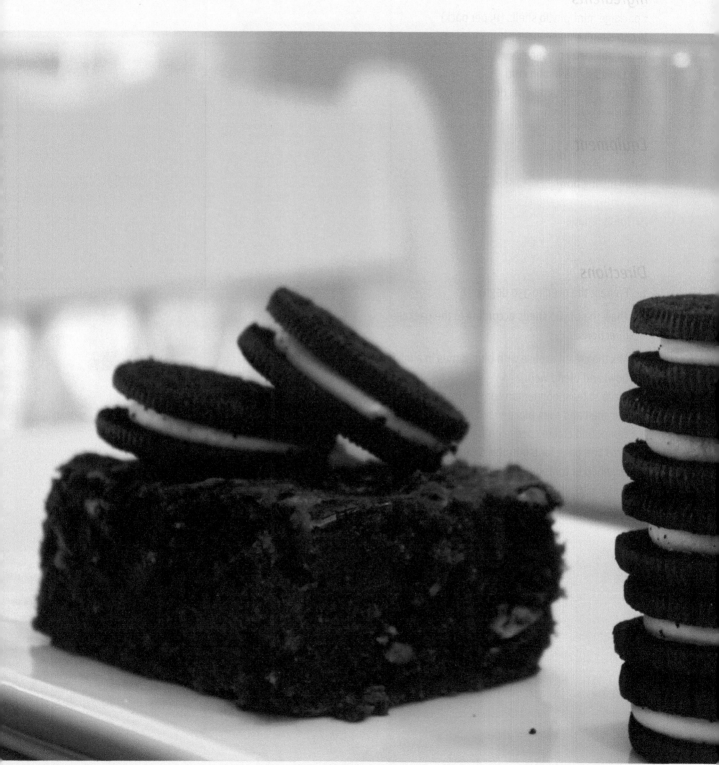

Servings: 6 - 8
Prep time: 10 minutes
Cooking time: 20 minutes
Cost: $6.11

Ingredients
10 Mint Crème Sandwich Cookies, crushed
Fudge brownie mix from a box
1 tablespoon peppermint extract
1 cup sour cream
Vegetable oil, water, and eggs as per package directions

Equipment
Mixing bowl
8 x 8 baking dish
Measuring cups & spoons

Directions
1. Preheat oven to 375 degrees F.

2. In a large mixing bowl, combine all the ingredients.
   You can use your hands (your best cooking tools!)
   to crush the cookies into the batter.
   Mix vigorously until everything is blended.

3. For thick, moist brownies, pour into an 8 x 8
   cooking dish and bake as per package directions.

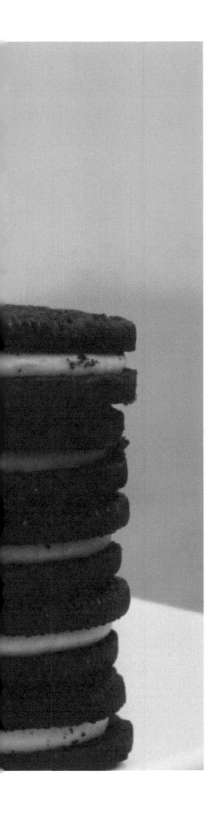

BANANA CHOCOLATE TARTS

Have you ever had bananas that are just about to go bad—at the perfect stage for banana bread? The following recipe is a great way to use those bananas you otherwise might throw out or put in the compost. It is not only delicious but also incredibly easy! It takes only 10 minutes to assemble the tarts and 25 minutes to cook them!

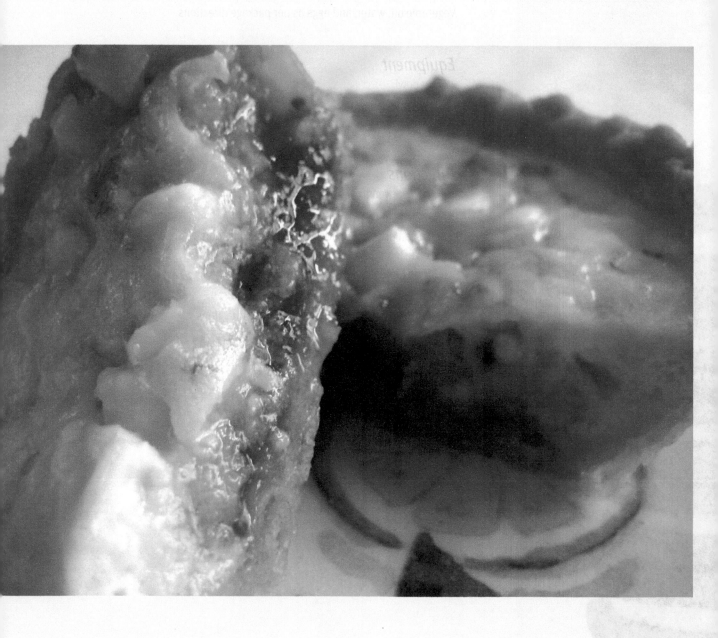

Servings: 8
Prep time: 10 minutes
Cooking time: 30 minutes
Cost: $6.03

Ingredients

1 package of 8 pastry shells * the pastry shells come in aluminum baking dishes
2 ripe bananas
4 teaspoons fig spread
½ cup white chocolate chips
½ cup cream or half and half
1 egg
½ teaspoon vanilla
¼ teaspoon salt

Equipment

2 small mixing bowls
Baking sheet
Measuring cups & spoons
Parchment paper (optional)

Directions

1. Preheat the oven to 350 degrees F.

2. In a small mixing bowl, mash the ripe bananas with a fork until smooth.

3. In another small mixing bowl, mix the cream, egg, vanilla, and salt (either a whisk or fork will work well).
   Secret tip: this is the same base used in quiche but sweet ingredients have been substituted.
   Separate and thaw the pastry shells according to the package directions.
   Place ½ teaspoon of the fig spread on the bottom of each pastry shell, followed by the 1 tablespoon of the mashed bananas, then 1 tablespoon of chocolate chips.
   Pour the custard mixture into the shells until it comes just to the top.
   Place the shells on a baking sheet and bake for 25 to 30 minutes until the custard is set.
   (It will be firm when touched.)

MASCARPONE COOKIE SANDWICHES

A creative alternative to the ice cream sandwich. Our mascarpone cookie sandwiches are very light and refreshing. If you're using fresh lime, lime zest sprinkled over the finished cookies makes for a beautiful presentation. You'll be amazed by how quick and easy this decadent treat can be.

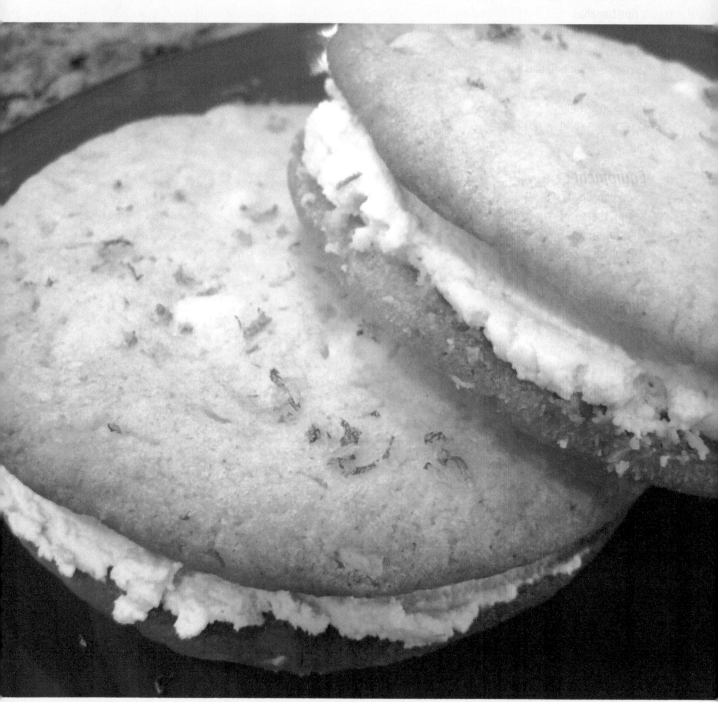

Servings: 5 - 6
Prep time: 10 minutes
Cooking time: 12 minutes
Cost: $10.71

Ingredients for the cookies

17.5 oz. bag of sugar cookie mix
1 egg
1 stick of unsalted butter
½ cup white chocolate chips
1 teaspoon almond extract
1 tablespoon orange juice
2 teaspoons lime juice

Ingredients for the filling

8 oz. mascarpone cheese (at room temperature)
1 teaspoon almond extract
1 teaspoon lime juice

Equipment

Mixing bowls (2)
Baking sheet
Ice cream scoop (optional)
Parchment paper (optional)

Directions

1. Leave the mascarpone cheese and butter on the counter for 1-2 hours to soften. Alternatively, you can microwave the butter, with or without the wrapper, for 12 seconds to soften.

2. Preheat the oven to 375 degrees F.

3. Mix the cookie ingredients in a bowl. Using an ice cream scoop, take a level scoop of batter and place on a baking sheet. You should get 10-12 cookies from this recipe to make 5 to 6 sandwiches. Bake for 11-12 minutes, until lightly brown. Let the cookies cool completely.

4. For the filling, mix the mascarpone with almond and lime. Spread 2 tablespoons of the filling over half the cookies and make a sandwich.

Chocolate Raspberry Custard

Use any chocolate you like in this recipe. Many of the chocolate bars in the baking aisle of the supermarket come in 4 oz size. This would be a great dessert to make for a fund raiser—at $1.25 per tart cost you could sell them easily for $2.50 and make 50% profit for your charity.

Servings: 8
Prep time: 5 minutes
Cooking time: 30 minutes
Cost: $10.06

Ingredients
4 oz. dark chocolate
4 oz. milk chocolate
3 tablespoons seedless raspberry preserves
1 cup heavy cream
2 eggs
Pinch of salt
8 mini pastry shells (comes in a box in the frozen
dessert section)

Equipment
Small saucepan
Mixing bowl
Measuring cups & spoons

Directions
1. Preheat the oven to 375 degrees F.

2. Thaw pastry shells according to package
   directions.

3. In a small saucepan, over medium-low heat,
   melt the chocolate with the cream and preserves.
   This takes about 5 minutes. Stir frequently.
   Turn off the heat.

4. In a small mixing bowl, whisk the eggs with
   a pinch of salt.
   Add 1-2 tablespoons of the warm chocolate
   mixture and whisk continuously.
   Repeat this process 2 more times.
   This will slowly bring up the temperature of
   the eggs so that they will not scramble
   (called tempering).
   Add back the egg mixture into the chocolate
   mixture and mix well.
   Pour into the mini pastry shells and bake
   for 25 minutes.

5. They are really delicious with fresh raspberries
   and whipped cream!

NEW ORLEANS BANANAS FOSTER CREPES

Our twist on a classic New Orleans dessert that was created at in the 1950's by a chef at Brennan's restaurant—a must stop for anyone visiting New Orleans! It was one of the best meals Ellen has ever had! Traditional bananas foster is made with rum and banana liqueur and served with ice cream. We've left out the alcohol. Please don't be intimidated by making crepes. They're basically just thin pancakes. You can fill them with sweet or savory ingredients. Try filling them with Brie, ham, and mushrooms—Mmm!

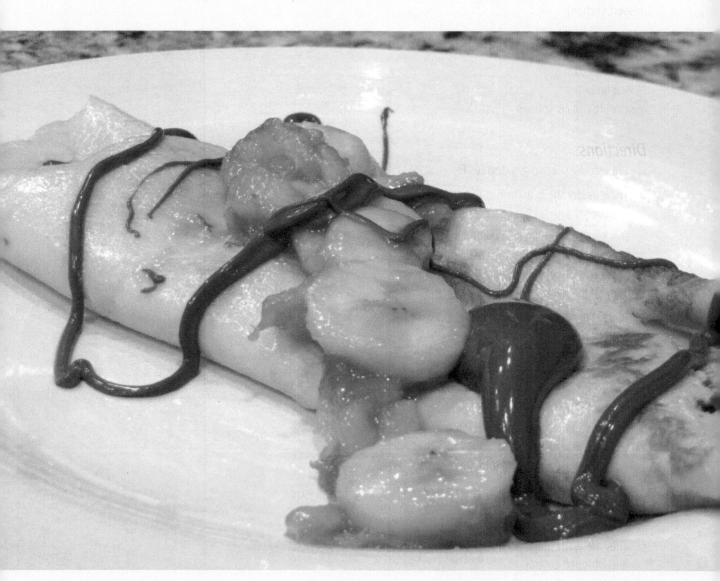

Crepe Ingredients

1 cup milk
¾ cup flour
3 lightly beaten eggs
1 tablespoon canola oil
1 pinch of salt
1/8 teaspoon ground nutmeg

Bananas Foster-Chocolate Hazelnut Sauce

2 cups melted chocolate hazelnut spread
1 teaspoon vanilla extract
6 – 8 bananas, thinly sliced
2 tablespoons brown sugar
2 tablespoons unsalted butter

Servings: 6 – 8
Prep time: 10 minutes
Cooking time: 10 minutes
Cost: $5.14

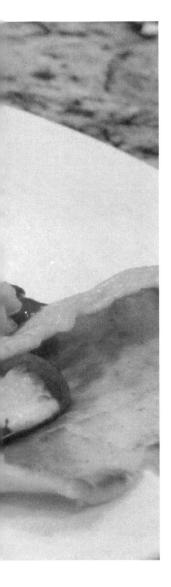

Equipment

1 nonstick sauté pan (for the crepes)
Medium size sauté pan
Mixing bowls
Microwave safe bowl (for melting the chocolate hazelnut spread)
Whisk
Measuring cups & spoons

Directions

For the crepe batter:

1. blend the flour, salt, and nutmeg in a medium-sized mixing bowl.
   In a separate bowl, lightly beat the eggs and then whisk them into the mixing bowl
   with the rest of the batter. Add the oil and continue to whisk.

2. Proceed to add the milk in slow increments, whisking until the batter thickens into
   a paste. Pour in the rest of the milk slowly and mix. You will notice that crepe batter
   is thinner than pancake batter.

To make the crepes:

1. preheat a nonstick sauté pan on medium heat for one minute and add butter until it
   melts and is distributed evenly.

2. Pour ¼ cup of batter into the middle of the pan. Remember to make sure it has
   spread over the surface of the pan and is sufficiently thin. Using a spatula, lift the side
   of the crepe after about half a minute. If it has browned, it's ready to be flipped over.
   Be very careful when flipping so that you don't break the crepe!

For the chocolate hazelnut sauce:

1. in a separate sauté pan over medium heat, melt 2 tablespoons of butter and the brown
   sugar and stir to combine, then add the banana slices and stir constantly for about
   2 minutes.

2. Add 1 teaspoon of vanilla extract and stir. Melt 2 cups of chocolate hazelnut sauce
   in a microwave-safe bowl for 1 minute on high, stirring after 30 seconds.
   Fold the bananas into the finished crepes, drizzle with sauce, and serve hot!

THYME TRUFFLES

Who says the Swiss have a monopoly on truffles? With our recipe, you can be your own budgeted gourmet chocolatier in a few short hours. Our savory truffles add an interesting and affordable element to your dessert. Use any ground herb or spice that strikes your fancy or leave out them out for a traditional truffle. Remember, the quality of the truffle is all about the quality of the chocolate. They also make a great holiday gift!

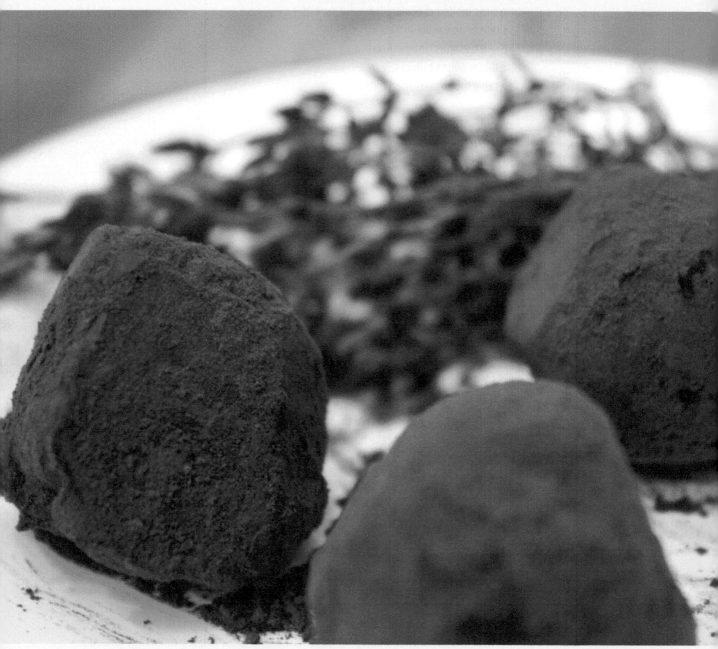

Servings: makes 20 truffles
Prep Time: 20 minutes
Inactive Prep Time: 1 hour
Cooking Time: 5 minutes
Cost: $6.25

Ingredients
8 oz. bittersweet chocolate
4 oz. (½ cup) cream
½ teaspoon ground thyme

Equipment
Small saucepan
Melon baller
Parchment paper
Whisk

Directions
1. In a small saucepan, bring the cream to a boil over medium heat, adding the ground thyme in as it warms up. Add the chocolate to the saucepan and mix until blended and smooth.
    The chocolate should take on a shiny, smooth consistency.

2. Allow it to cool in the fridge for 10 minutes, then remove and whisk vigorously with a wire whisk for 1 full minute. Cover and chill for 1 hour.

3. After the chocolate has cooled, scoop out with a small melon baller onto parchment paper.
    Roll the chocolate into balls.
    Be sure to have a cup of hot water on hand for dipping the scooper; this will make it easier for the chocolate to slide off.

4. When you are ready to serve, have a bowl with cocoa powder on hand nearby.
    Roll the truffles gently between your palms to attain a rounder shape; then cover them with cocoa powder and place on a plate.
    Fresh truffles can be kept in the fridge for two weeks.

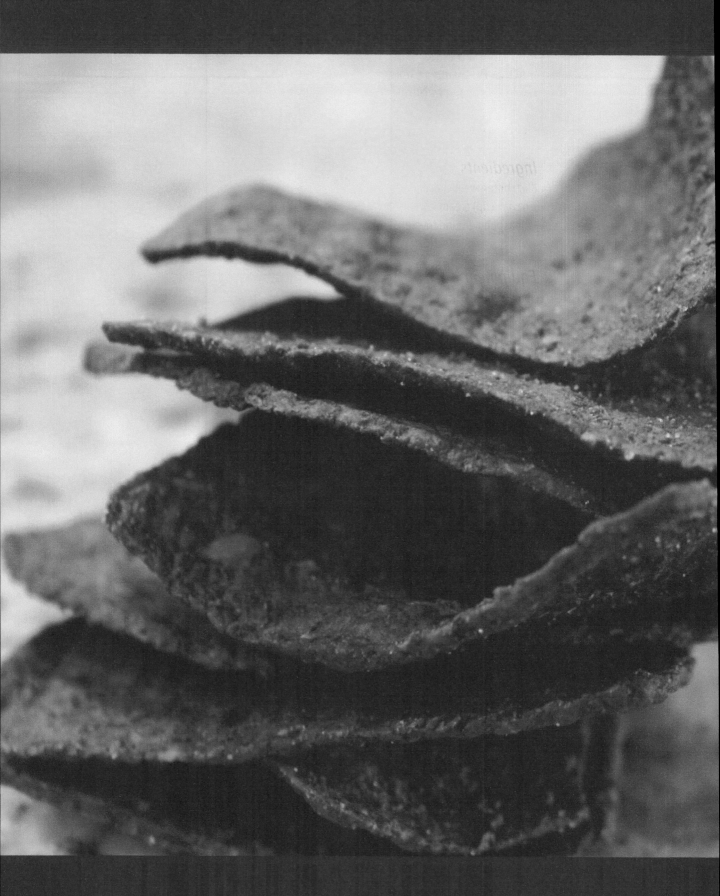

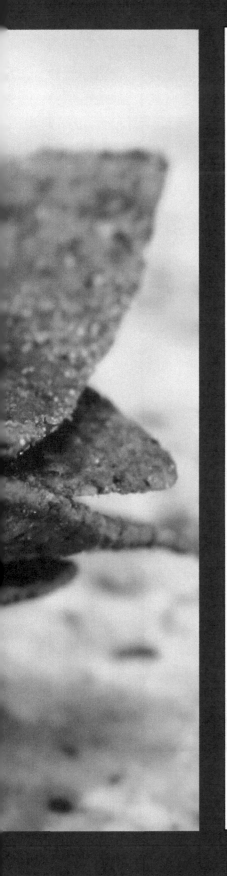

Mexican Arriba Bean Dip

3 a.m. Tricolore

40 Second Nachos

Tuna Avocado Boats

Sweet and Salty Cottage Cheese and Melon

A Study in Popcorn (Popcorn 3 ways)

Gourmet Fratbread

New Orleans Spicy White Bean and Garlic Dip

Parmesan Crisps

Sautéed Zucchini Bites

MEXICAN ARRIBA BEAN DIP

If you're looking for a healthy snack in the wee small hours of the morning and are fed up with spending all your money on take-out, try our bean dip! The refreshing flavors will refuel any tired student. Store in the fridge for a repeat performance the next night! Warm either in the oven or microwave.

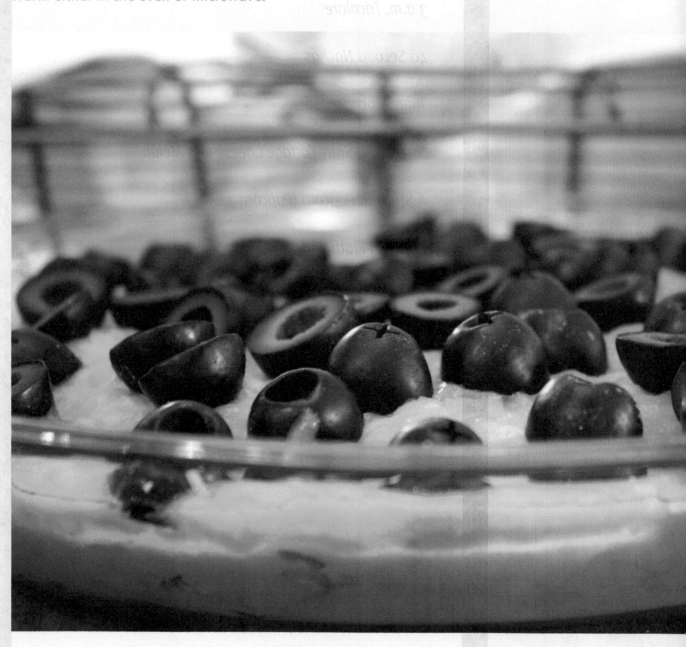

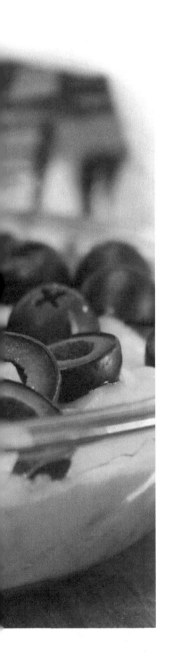

Servings: 8 - 10
Prep time: 5 minutes
Cook time: 5 – 10 minutes
Cost: $10.14

Ingredients

½ can jumbo pitted olives, 15.5 oz can, drained
15.5 oz. can whole kernel corn, drained
15.5 oz. can refried beans
8 oz. package of shredded cheese (your choice)
8 oz. sour cream
8 squirts of your favorite hot sauce for mild, 12 squirts
for a hot dip

Equipment

9 or 10 inch pie dish or large microwave-safe bowl for serving
Chopping knife
Mixing bowl

Directions

1. Preheat the oven at 375 degrees F.

2. Slice the olives in half. Mix the sour cream with the hot sauce in a mixing bowl.

3. This dish is all about layers. The first layer to go into the bowl will be the refried beans.

4. Next, apply the sour cream/hot sauce mixture.

5. After that, spread the can of corn over the mix, and then sprinkle the whole dish with the shredded cheese.

6. To finish, arrange the sliced olives on top and place in the oven for 8 to 10 minutes.

Alternatively, you can microwave for 5 minutes. Enjoy with tortilla chips! We recommend chips with a lime flavor for an extra zing.

3 A.M. TRICOLORE

It's about that time of night with no end in sight. To take a refreshing and healthy break from studies, treat yourself to our mozzarella bites. Hopefully, the colors of Italy will refuel you. Also great as an appetizer for guests.

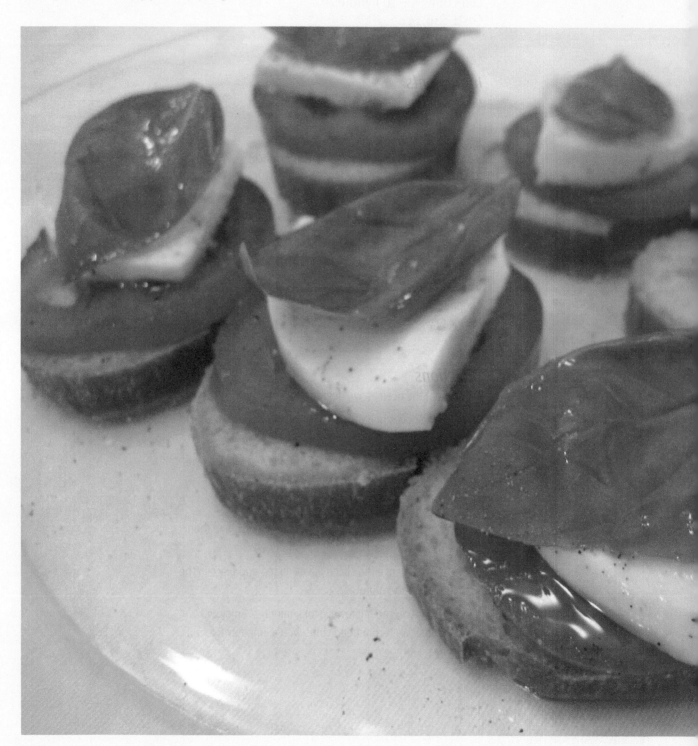

Servings: 6 - 8
Prep time: 10 minutes
Cook time: 0
Cost: $10.40

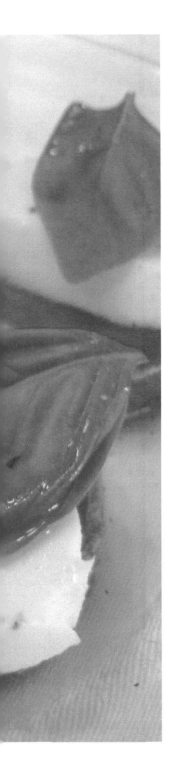

Ingredients
8 oz. block of fresh whole milk mozzarella cheese
3 ripe plum tomatoes
½ fresh French baguette (will give about 20 slices)
20 fresh basil leaves
Olive oil
Salt and pepper

Equipment
Serrated knife
Cutting board

Directions
Slice the block of mozzarella in to thin slices—you should get about 20 slices from an 8 ounce block. Slice the tomatoes into thin slices. You can use any type of tomato for this dish but the plum tomatoes are exactly the right size to top the baguette. Slice the baguette into ¼ inch slices (save the other half for fig and gorgonzola bites!). Layer as follows: tomato, mozzarella, basil. You'll want approximately one leaf of basil per piece of baguette, although leaf size may vary. Drizzle with olive, then sprinkle with salt and pepper to taste. Allora, easy bites anytime.

40 SECOND NACHOS

Yes, only 40 seconds—as long as you have a microwave. Don't fret if you do not have one—put the nachos in the oven at 350 degrees F for 5-6 minutes until the cheese is melted and you have an equally delicious snack.

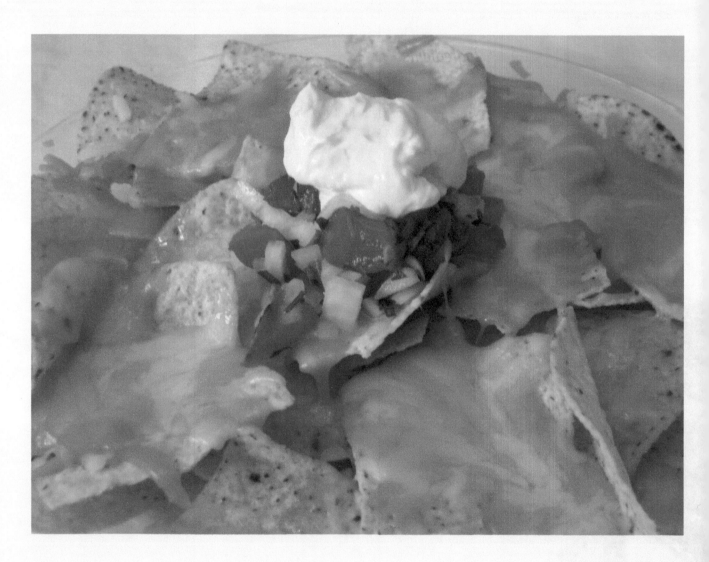

Servings: 2
Prep time: 5 minutes
Cooking time: 40 seconds
Cost: $4.08

Ingredients

2 handfuls corn tortilla chips
1 cup Monterey jack cheese/cheddar cheese (comes in packages)
2 dollops sour cream

Salsa Ingredients

1 large ripe tomato, diced
½ large white onion, diced
¼ cup fresh cilantro, chopped
1 tablespoon lemon juice
1 tablespoon lime juice
½ teaspoon salt

Equipment

Microwave safe dinner plate
Cutting board & paring knife
Measuring cups & spoons

Directions

1. Place the tortilla chips on a microwave safe, dinner-size plate and generously sprinkle with your favorite cheese (we recommend Monterey Jack/Cheddar combo).

2. Before putting the nachos into the microwave, dice the tomato and onion. Chop up the cilantro and mix with the rest of the salsa ingredients in a small bowl.

3. Microwave the chips and cheese. Remove, cover with the salsa and sour cream, and serve hot! We've discovered that 40 seconds is the perfect time frame (when a microwave is set to high) for maintaining the crispiness of the chips while thoroughly melting the cheese. Some microwaves may vary on power, so check after 30 seconds to make sure the cheese doesn't begin to brown.

TUNA AVOCADO BOATS

Yet another healthy way to cure the late-night munchies.
Avocado is a universal vessel, so you can substitute any kind of
salad for the tuna if it's not your favorite fish.

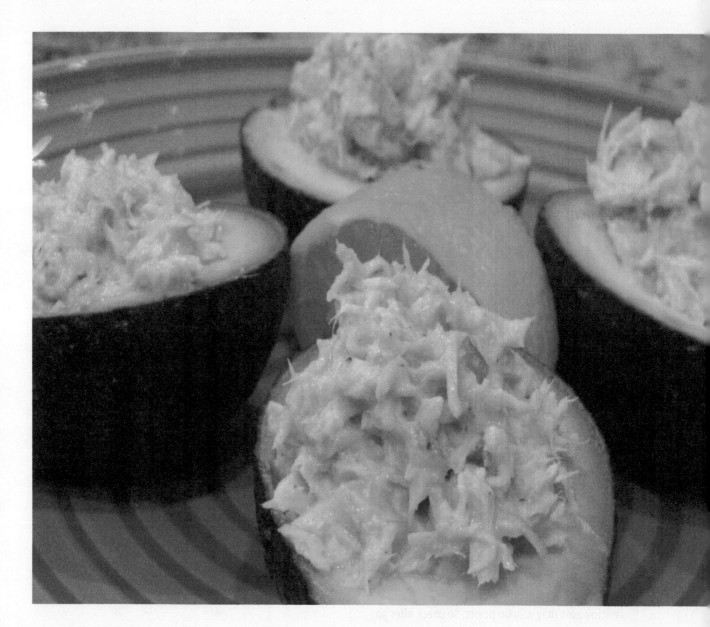

Servings: 4
Prep time: 8 minutes
Cooking time: 0
Cost: $5.70

Ingredients

3 ripe avocados
2 cans of dolphin-safe water based tuna
2 teaspoons sweet relish
1 heaping tablespoon of mayonnaise
1 teaspoon of balsamic vinegar
1 teaspoon of lemon juice
½ teaspoon of Dijon mustard
¼ teaspoon of ground black pepper

Equipment

Paring knife
Spoon
Can opener
Measuring spoons

Directions

1. Halve the avocados and carefully remove the pits with a spoon. Try to preserve the impression left by the pit, because you will be putting the tuna salad in there.

2. Empty the cans of tuna into the mixing bowl.
   Add in the rest of the ingredients as listed above and mix thoroughly with a fork.
   When you are finished, scoop up the salad and place it into the craters left by the pit of the avocado.

SWEET AND SALTY COTTAGE CHEESE AND MELON

Choose this for your midnight snack and you'll have amazing energy for finishing that paper or studying for a morning exam. This dish features a delightful balance of succulent sweetness from the honey and melon and saltiness from the cheese. You won't even realize you're eating a healthy snack!

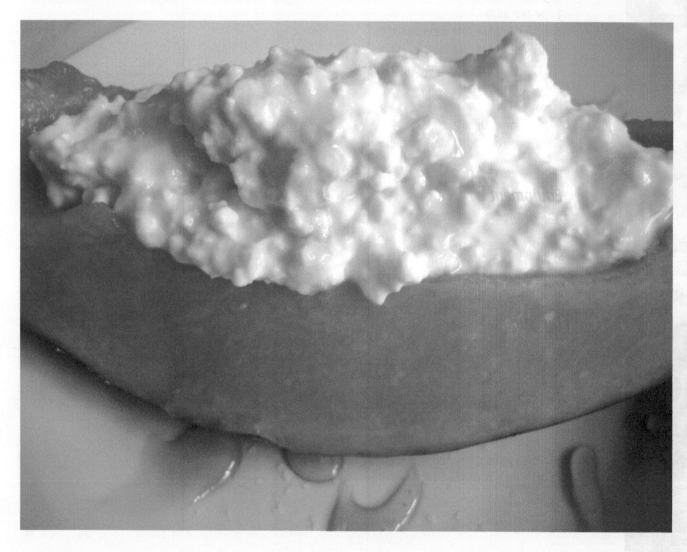

Servings: 4
Prep time: 5 minutes
Cooking time: 0 minutes
Cost: $5.50

Ingredients

1 cantaloupe (a sweet melon)
2 cups cottage cheese
Honey
Salt

Equipment

Knife to slice melon
Measuring cup

Directions

1. Cut the melon in half if serving 2 or in quarters if serving 4. Scoop out the seeds.

2. Place ½ cup cottage cheese on top of the melon slice.

3. Drizzle with honey and a pinch of salt.

A STUDY IN POPCORN (POPCORN 3 WAYS)

Here's a gourmet cure for your salty and sweet cravings. Whether you're watching a movie with friends or up late studying, you'll be sure to satisfy any kind of flavor craving with our spiced up popcorn recipes.

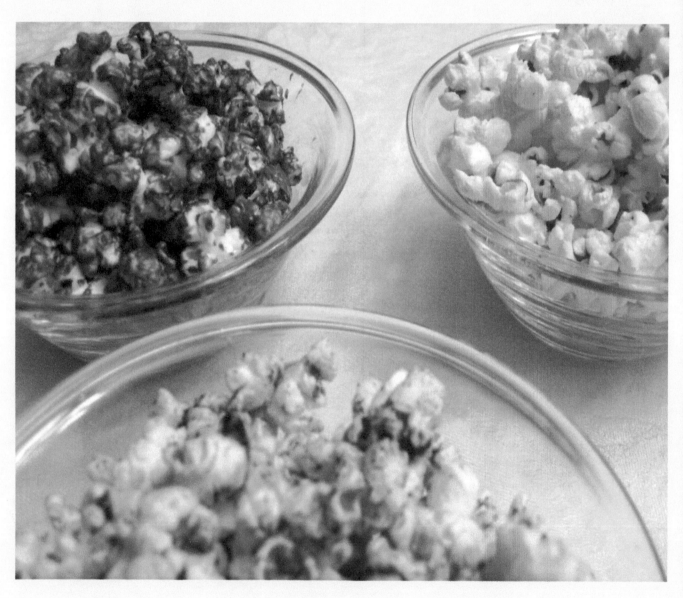

Servings: 4 per batch
Prep time: 5 minutes per batch
Cook time: 3-5 minutes per batch
Cost: Garlic: $3.73
          Chocolate: $2.70
          Cajun: $1.83
          Total: $8.26

I. Garlicky Cheese Popcorn
Ingredients
Popcorn (1 package or ½ cup raw kernels)
½ cup grated Parmesan (4 tablespoons)
1 tablespoon garlic powder
1 tablespoon salt
4 tablespoons melted, unsalted butter (1/2 stick)

Directions
N. B.: if you're using popcorn from a container and not prepackaged, follow the instructions for stove popping on the side of the container. Generally, ½ cup of raw kernels should serve about 5 people. If your butter is salted, eliminate the salt from the recipe.

Cook the popcorn as per package directions. Melt the butter in a microwave-safe dish until melted (30 seconds). Pour the butter over your popcorn and mix thoroughly. Then sprinkle the Parmesan, salt, and garlic powder over the popcorn. Toss until mixed well and serve hot!

II. White Chocolate Hazelnut Popcorn
Ingredients
Popcorn (1 package or ½ cup raw kernels)
½ cup melted chocolate hazelnut spread
½ cup melted white chocolate chips

Directions
Cook the popcorn as per package directions. Melt the chocolate spread and white chocolate chips in separate microwave-safe bowls: 1-½ minutes for the white chips and 1 minute for the chocolate spread. It is easiest to stir and drizzle the chocolate sauce over the popcorn with a standard dinner knife. Sprinkle with sea salt for a different kind of twist. Refrigerate your leftover chocolate sauce for use the next day.

III. Cajun Sugar Popcorn
Ingredients
Popcorn (1 package or ½ cup raw kernels)
4 tablespoons melted unsalted butter
1 tablespoon ancho chile powder
1 teaspoon cinnamon
1 teaspoon salt

Directions
N. B. If you're using salted butter, remove the salt from the recipe.

Cook the popcorn as per package direction. Melt the butter for 30 seconds in the microwave. Add the ancho chile powder and cinnamon to the butter and mix. Drizzle over the popcorn 3 teaspoons at a time and mix thoroughly before drizzling again. Sprinkle with 2 teaspoons of salt as a finishing touch.

GOURMET FRATBREAD

You may not want to share this one!

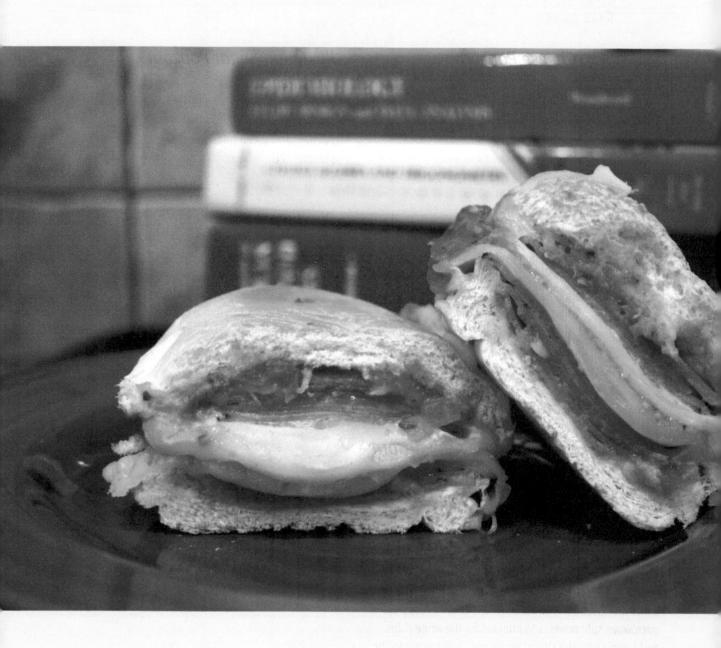

Servings: 1 - 2
Prep time: 5 minutes
Cooking time: 10 minutes
Cost: $4.55

Ingredients

2 slices salami
2 slices sandwich-size pepperoni
2 slices ham
2 slices mozzarella cheese
2 teaspoons Parmesan cheese (shredded or grated)
4 tablespoons marinara sauce
2 teaspoons Dijon mustard (any mustard you have in the fridge will work)
1 hamburger bun or sliced Italian loaf

Equipment

Baking sheet
Measuring spoons

Directions

Slice a hoagie roll, hamburger bun, or any type of bread into halves and layer
the following ingredients in this order on each half:

1. 2 tablespoons marinara sauce
2. 2 slices of salami
3. 2 slices of pepperoni (sandwich size--use 5-6 if you have the small rounds)
4. 2 slices of ham
5. 1 teaspoon Dijon mustard
6. 2 slices of sliced deli style mozzarella cheese
7. 2 tablespoons marinara sauce
8. 2 teaspoons Parmesan cheese

This is basically a leftover baked open-face sandwich—put on whatever is
left in your fridge that you want to use up or have a craving for. Bake at 400
degrees F for 10 minutes. You can share it or save it all for yourself.

You can also make a mile-high sandwich by placing the halves together.

NEW ORLEANS SPICY WHITE BEAN AND GARLIC DIP

This is a great dip for a picnic—none of the ingredients is perishable.
This dip is wonderful with our toasted cumin pita chips.

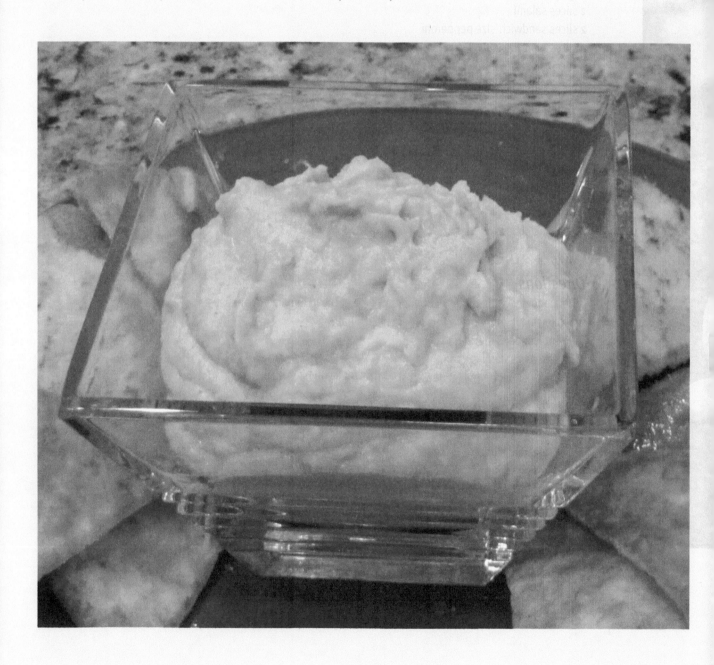

Servings: 6 - 8
Prep time: 3 minute
Cooking time: 0 minutes
Cost: $1.37

Ingredients

15 oz. can of cannellini beans
5 tablespoons olive oil
1 tablespoon garlic paste
¼ teaspoon salt
¼ teaspoon cayenne pepper for mild, ½ teaspoon for spicy

Equipment

2 cup food processor

Directions

Blend all the ingredients in a food processor until smooth.
Serve with tortilla chips or pita bread.

PARMESAN CRISPS

If you're in a salty mood at midnight these will completely satisfy your craving. We also serve these with our Caesar salad. If you're doing the low-carb thing, these are a fantastic snack.

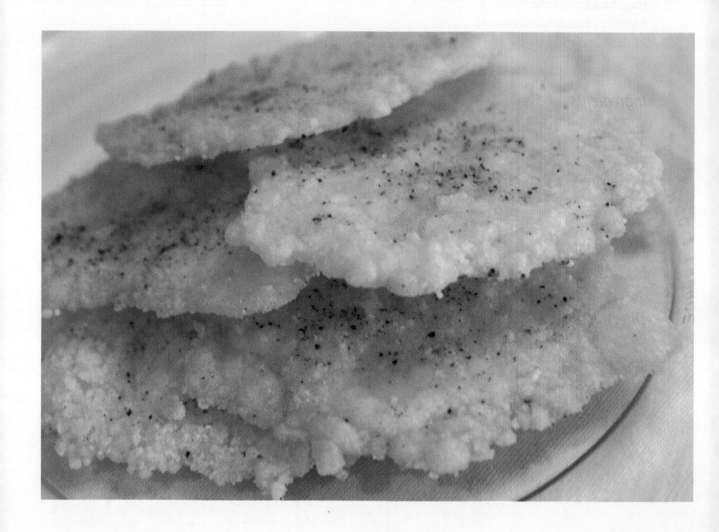

Servings: 4
Prep time: 5 minutes
Cooking time: 5 minutes
Cost: $2.00

Ingredients

1 cup Parmesan cheese
Ground black pepper

Equipment

Baking sheet

Directions

1. Mound 1 tablespoon of Parmesan on a baking sheet and press down the center with the spoon.

2. Place in a 400 degree F oven for 5 minutes.

3. Sprinkle with pepper.

SAUTÉED ZUCCHINI BITES

Tired of raw vegetables? Here's an excellent way to eat healthily and still satisfy your tatsebuds. These little zucchini bites are quick, easy, and delicious. Perfect for unexpected guests or for the 2 a.m. studying hunger attack, they're a simple way to add flair to your day.

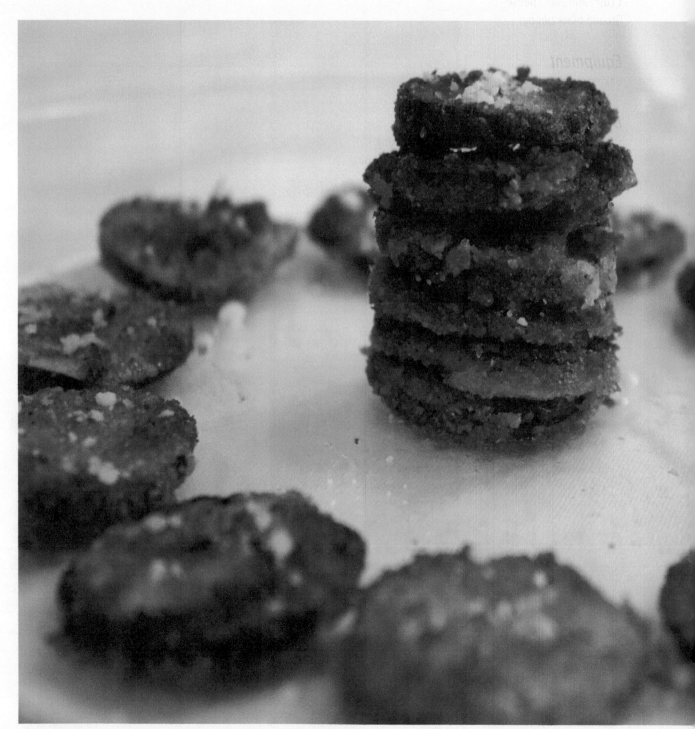

Servings: 4
Prep time: 10 minutes
Cooking time: 5 minutes
Cost: $2.61

Ingredients
2 large eggs, beaten
1/8 teaspoon cayenne pepper
¼ teaspoon salt
1 teaspoon garlic paste
¼ cup olive oil
1 cup bread crumbs
¼ cup Parmesan cheese
Pinch of salt
1 zucchini, thinly sliced

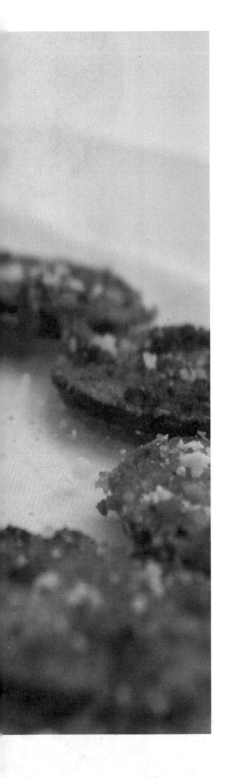

Equipment
Cutting board
Chopping knife
Whisk (optional)
Sauté pan
3 bowls
Spatula
Measuring cups & spoons

Directions
1. Slice the zucchini into ½ inch thick rounds.
   Heat the sauté pan to medium-low heat with
   1 tablespoon of olive oil and the garlic paste.

2. In a bowl, whisk the eggs. In a separate bowl m
   mix the breadcrumbs, Parmesan cheese, salt,
   and cayenne.

3. Coat the slices of zucchini with olive oil, then
   dip in the egg mixture and coat thoroughly,
   then cover completely in the breadcrumb mixture.
   Place gingerly into the sauté pan and sauté for
   about 1 – 2 minutes per side.

4. Remove with a spatula and place on a paper towel
   or napkin to let the excess oil drain.
   Salt immediately.

5. Serve warm and crispy!

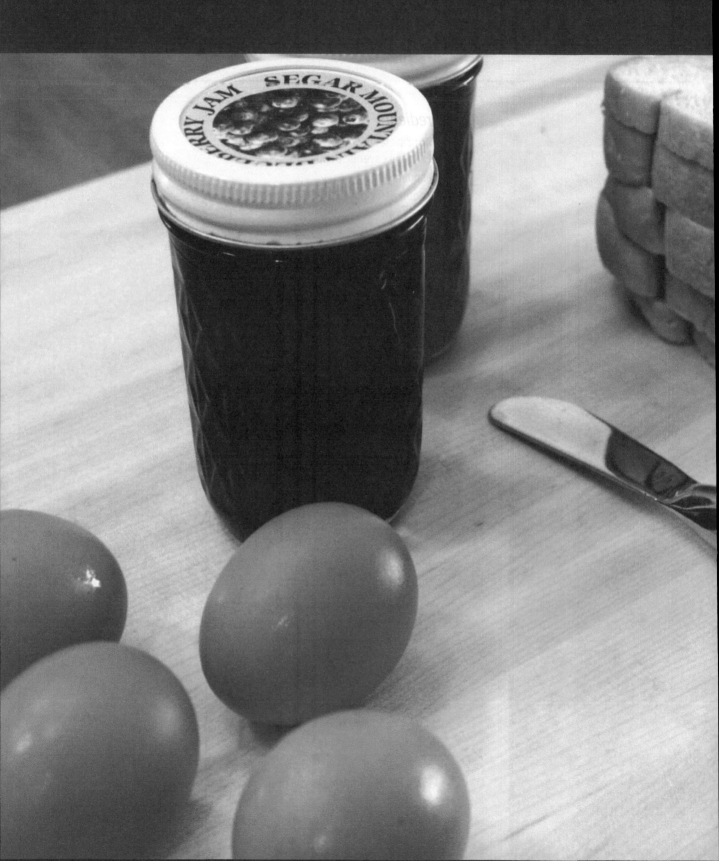

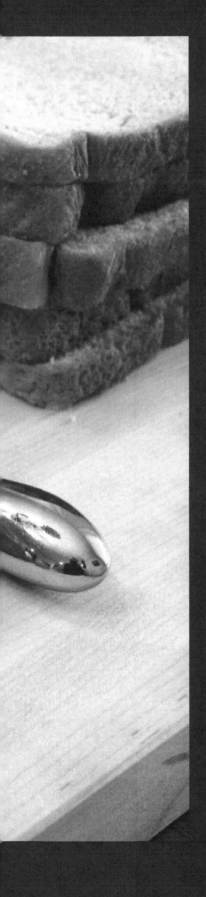

Blanc et Bleu Pancakes

California Scramble

Sweet and Savory Cream Cheese Trio

Fettuccini Alfredo Frittata

Egg Salad over Flatbread

New Orleans Eggs Benedict

Memphis French Toast Sandwich

Omelet Provençal for One

Baja Breakfast Bonanza

BLANC ET BLEU PANCAKES

Whether you're cooking for yourself or gathering friends for a leisurely brunch, these pancakes will be sure to satisfy all palates present. We recommend using blueberry preserves, but you can substitute raspberry, cherry, or any other type of fruit that suits your taste buds. You can vary this recipe based on your personal preferences. Substitute savory flavors for sweet such as ham and cheese or corn and black beans. Dark chocolate with raspberry preserves is one of our favorite combinations.

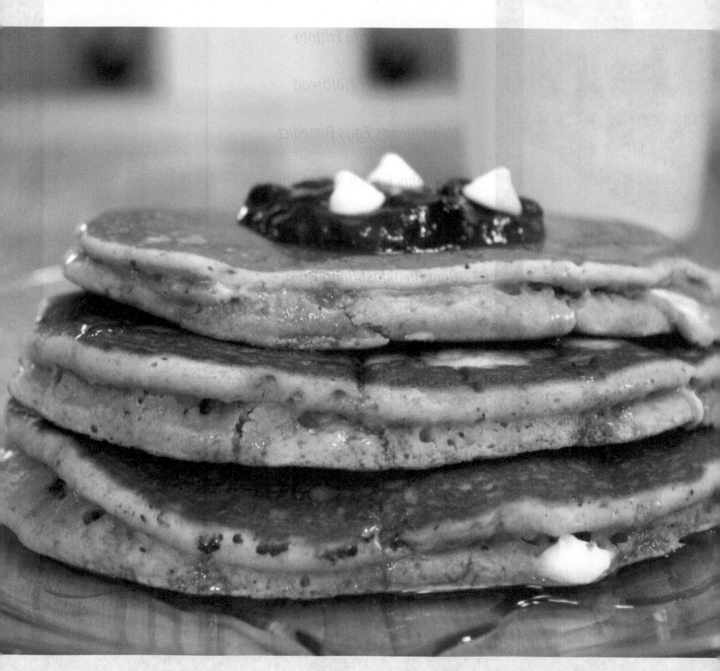

Servings: makes 8-9 pancakes
Prep time: 5 minutes
Cooking time: 2 - 4 minutes per
pancake
Cost: $2.60

Ingredients

2 ½ cups pancake mix
1 cup milk
2 eggs
2 heaping tablespoons blueberry preserves
¾ cups white chocolate morsels
1 teaspoon vegetable oil per 2 pancakes

Equipment

Large sauté pan
Spatula
Mixing bowl
Measuring cups & spoons (use the 1/2 cup measure for pouring
pancakes into the pan)

Directions

1. Pour the pancake mix, milk and eggs into a
   large mixing bowl. Mix thoroughly, then add the blueberry
   preserves and the white chocolate morsels and stir.

2. Set the stovetop to medium-low heat.
   When making pancakes, it is especially important to test
   that the pan has properly heated.
   You can do so by spattering water on the surface of the
   metal. If it bubbles, the pan has heated sufficiently
   (the process should take about 2 minutes).
   Pour 1 teaspoon of oil into the pan and make
   sure that it has spread evenly.
   Our old family trick is to use a folded paper towel to
   spread the oil.
   You can cook 2 pancakes with each teaspoon of oil.
   You will need to add another teaspoon after every
   2 pancakes.

3. When the pan is ready, pour 1/2 cup of batter into it
   and cook for about 1 – 2 minutes on each side.
   It is ready to flip when the top is covered with bubbles
   and when the underside is a light brown color.
   Place a dollop of blueberry preserves on top of your
   pancake stack and finish with maple syrup.

CALIFORNIA SCRAMBLE

Add a spicy touch of the Pacific to your Saturday morning. We recommend using goat cheese crumbles (available in 4 oz. packages), but a large stick of goat cheese works well too.

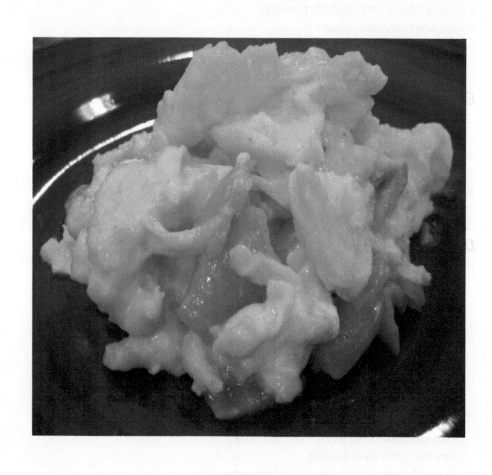

Serves: 4 - 6
Prep time: 10 minutes
Cooking time: 5 minutes
Price: $7.54

Ingredients

12 eggs
4 tablespoons of milk or cream
1/8 teaspoon of cayenne pepper
5 tablespoons of crumbled goat cheese (half of a 4 oz package)
1 tablespoon of unsalted butter
2 oz. of smoked salmon (comes in 4 oz. packages)

Equipment

Large mixing bowl
Medium or large sauté pan
Fork or spatula
Whisk
Paring knife
Mixing bowl
Measuring spoons

Directions

1. Crack all the eggs into a large mixing bowl.
   Whisk until the yolks have broken, and the eggs are evenly yellow.
   Add the milk and cayenne and whisk again.

2. Open the package of smoked salmon and use your hands (or a knife) to separate 2 oz. (about half the normal package size).
   Break the salmon into smaller pieces using either a knife or your hands.

3. Set the stove to medium-low heat and melt 1 tablespoon of butter.
   Once the butter has melted, pour in the eggs.
   Using a fork or spatula, gently move the eggs around the pan as the eggs are cooking; otherwise, you might end up with an omelet!
   It will take about 5 minutes for the eggs to cook.

4. Once the eggs have cooked, turn off the heat, add the salmon and goat cheese, and mix.

Sweet and Savory Cream Cheese Trio

You'll marvel at the amazing ease of putting together a breakfast buffet with pizzazz. If you make our 3 cream cheese spreads—smoked salmon, blueberry, and carrot-raisin—and serve them with a variety of muffins and breads, you'll be a star!

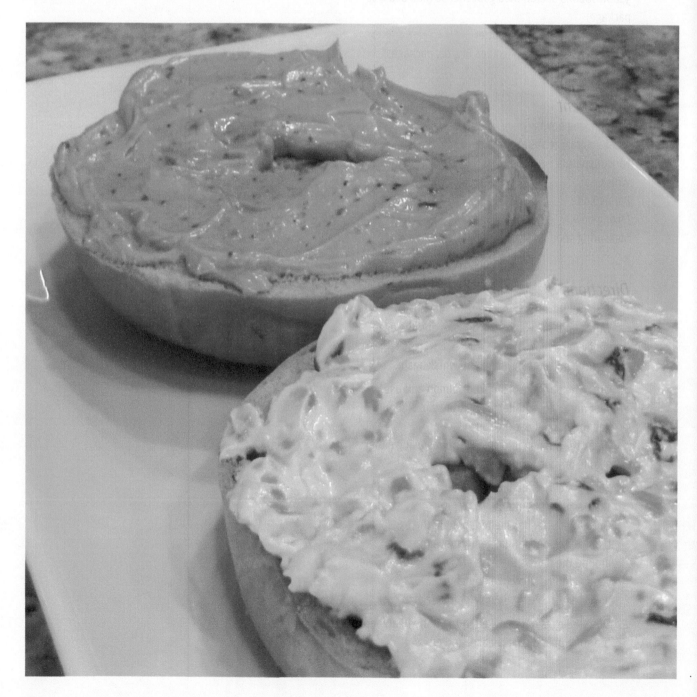

Carrot Raisin Cream Cheese Spread

Servings: 4 - 6
Prep time: 1 minute
Cost: $3.01

Ingredients

8 oz. package cream cheese
½ cup shredded carrots
¼ cup of golden or dark raisins
1 tablespoon brown sugar (light or dark)

Equipment

2 cup food processor (optional)
Measuring cups & spoons

Directions

1. Let the cream cheese sit on the counter for 1-2 hours to soften.

2. Mix the cream cheese and brown sugar in a food processor.

3. Fold in the carrots and raisins with a spoon and serve with your favorite toasted bread. You can also do this by hand.

Blueberry Cream Cheese Spread

Servings: 4 - 6
Prep time: 1 minute
Cost: $3.19

Ingredients

8 oz. package cream cheese
3 tablespoons blueberry preserves

Equipment

2-cup food processor (optional)
Measuring spoons

Directions

1. Let the cream cheese sit on the counter for 1-2 hours to soften.

2. Mix the cream cheese and preserves in a food processor until smooth.

3. Serve over toasted bagels or toast.

* You can also do this by hand, mixing the cream cheese and blueberries thoroughly and even serve from the same bowl.

Smoked Salmon Cream Cheese Spread

Servings: 4 - 6
Prep time: 1 minute
Cost: $ 5.25

Ingredients

2 oz. of smoked salmon (comes in 4 oz. packages)
8 oz. cream cheese
¼ cup of sour cream
2 tablespoons of lemon juice
¼ teaspoon of black pepper

Equipment

2 cup food processor
Measuring cups & spoons

Directions

1. Blend all the ingredients in a food processor until you reach your desired consistency.
   For a chunkier dip you could cut the smoked salmon into small pieces and mix all ingredients by hand.

2. Serve with toast or bagels. You can make a New York City bagel sandwich by layering the smoked salmon spread on a bagel and topping with sliced red onion and tomato.
   It's wonderful!

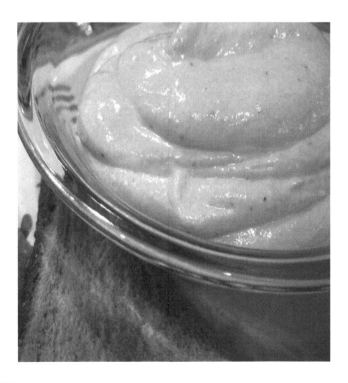

FETTUCCINI ALFREDO FRITTATA

Cooking for a large crowd? Need to get rid of a dozen eggs in a hurry?
You'll be able to satisfy multiple palates with our Sunday morning frittata.
The best thing about a frittata recipe is that you can substitute whatever ingredients
you choose, building on our basic steps.

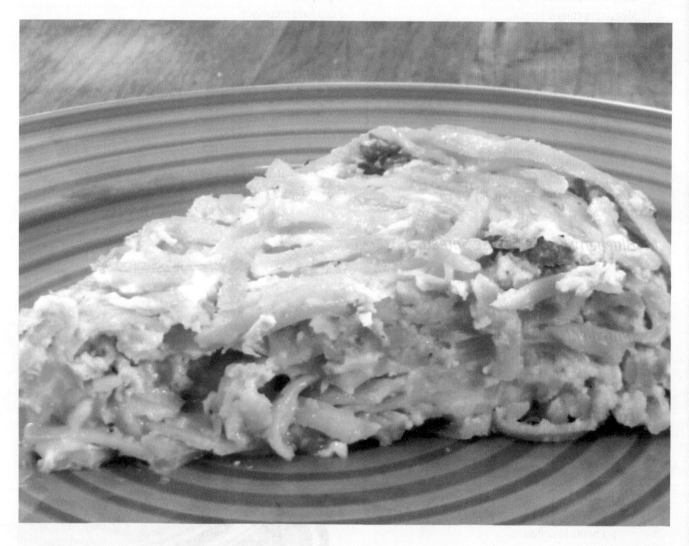

Servings: 6 - 8
Prep time: 10 minutes
Cooking time: 20 minutes
Cost: $14.79

Ingredients

12 eggs
16 oz. package fettuccini
2 cups heavy cream
1 cup grated Parmesan
8 oz. package mushrooms, sliced
½ pound deli ham
2 tablespoons unsalted butter
2 tablespoons olive oil
1 teaspoon salt
½ teaspoon ground black pepper
¼ teaspoon ground nutmeg

Equipment

Pasta pot
Oven-safe large sauté pan
Cutting board & paring knife
Measuring cups & spoons
Mixing bowl
Whisk
Spatula

Directions

1. Preheat the oven to 425 degrees F.

2. Boil water in a large pasta pot.
   When the water comes to a boil, add 2 tablespoons of salt and then the pasta.
   Cook for approximately four minutes less than the package directions indicate, leaving it slightly al dente. The pasta will be cooking on the stove and in the oven, so don't worry about the texture just yet.

3. In a mixing bowl, whisk the eggs and add 1 teaspoon of salt and ½ teaspoon of pepper, ¼ teaspoon ground nutmeg, and set aside.
   As a rule, always use nutmeg in your cream sauces.

4. While the pasta is boiling, you can chop up the mushrooms and ham into good-sized chunks.
   Heat an oven-safe large sauté pan over medium-high heat with butter and olive oil.
   Add the mushrooms and ham and cook for 4 minutes.
   Then add the pasta, cream, and Parmesan and reduce the heat to medium.
   Toss to coat the pasta with the cream sauce.

5. Pour egg mixture over the pasta.
   Cook for about 5 minutes over medium heat, until the bottom of the mixture has begun to solidify.
   Put the sauté pan directly into the preheated oven and cook for 10 minutes.
   Slice like a pizza and serve alone or with a green salad.

EGG SALAD OVER FLATBREAD

Ever feel caught between breakfast and lunch?
Our flatbread egg salad sandwich will be a delicious
compromise. Also great for a late-night snack.

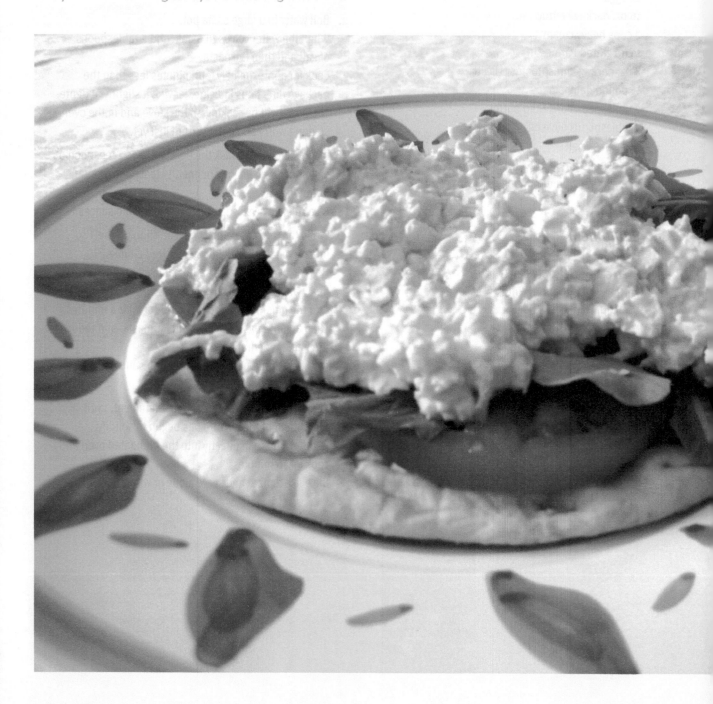

Servings: 4
Prep time: 15 minutes
Cook time: 12 minutes
Cost: $8.56

Ingredients

8 hard boiled eggs
4 pieces flatbread
2 cups of arugula
2 tomatoes, sliced
8 slices Munster cheese
3 tablespoons mayonnaise
1 tablespoon Dijon mustard
1 tablespoon shredded Parmesan cheese
1 teaspoon salt
¼ teaspoon black pepper
3 squirts your favorite hot sauce
Olive oil, salt, and pepper to taste over finished sandwich

Equipment

Saucepan for boiling eggs
Mixing bowl

Directions

1. Hard boil the eggs by placing in a saucepan in cold water;
   enough to just cover the eggs, and bring to a boil then reduce
   to medium-low heat for 10 minutes.
   Let cool and peel.

2. Place eggs in a mixing bowl and mash with a fork.

3. Add the mayo, mustard, cheese, salt, pepper, and hot
   sauce and mix well.
   Drizzle olive oil (about 1 teaspoon) over the flatbread; place
   2 slices of Munster cheese (evenly distributed over the bread)
   on each piece of flat bread, then toast in a toaster or under
   the broiler until the cheese has melted.
   Make sure to keep a vigilant eye on the cheese; it burns quickly!

4. Place three slices of a large, ripe tomato on each slice of
   flatbread and sprinkle with salt and pepper to taste, then
   drizzle with olive oil.

5. Place a bed of arugula on each piece of bread, cover with the
   egg salad (the equivalent of about 2 eggs per person), and
   serve hot!
   Depending on the size of the flatbread, it might be easier to cut
   into halves or quarters and eat by hand or with a fork and knife.

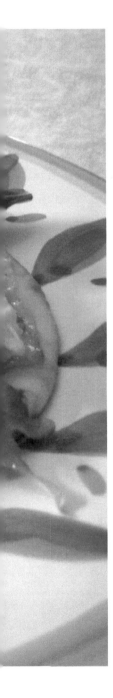

NEW ORLEANS EGGS BENEDICT

We've created a fusion of flavors to add Louisiana flair to the favorite brunch staple, Eggs Benedict. Instead of going to a diner, dine in with friends while helping yourselves to a gourmet recipe with a maritime kick.

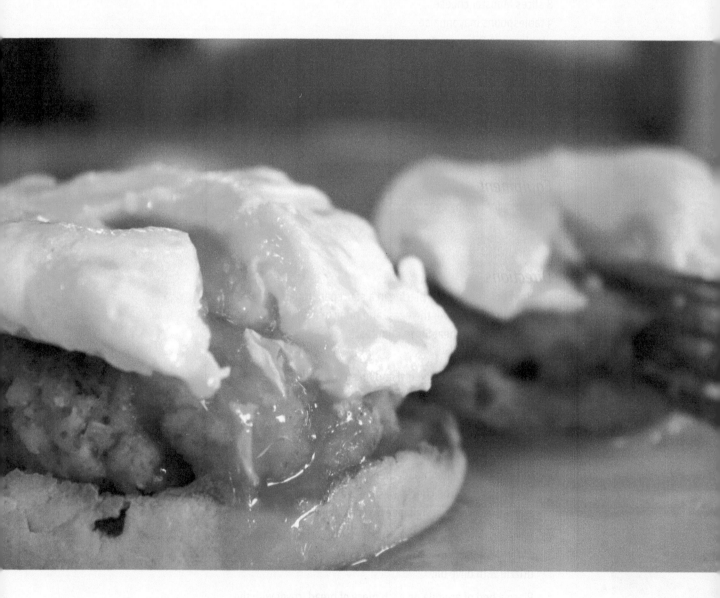

Servings: 6
Prep time: 15 minutes
Cooking time: 20 minutes
Cost: $10.28

Ingredients
6 English muffins
1 + 12 eggs
1 pound shrimp (pre-cooked, peeled and
    deveined, fresh or frozen)
1 green onion (scallion), finely chopped
¼ teaspoon cayenne pepper
1 teaspoon lime juice
¾ cup breadcrumbs
2 tablespoons vegetable oil
1 teaspoon salt
1 tablespoon white vinegar
    (for the poaching water)
Hollandaise sauce (see below)

Hollandaise Sauce Ingredients
3 egg yolks
1 stick of unsalted butter
2 teaspoons lemon juice
½ teaspoon salt

Equipment
Sauté pan x 2 (one for poaching the eggs and
    one for the shrimp patties)
Small saucepan for melting the butter
    (or microwave for 45 seconds)
Slotted spoon for poached eggs
Spatula
Measuring cups & spoons
Blender (optional)
Food processor (optional)

Directions
Shrimp patties:
Puree the shrimp in a food processor (if you don't have a food processor, you can chop the shrimp into small pieces). Put the pureed shrimp in a mixing bowl and add the green onion, 1 egg, breadcrumbs, lime juice, cayenne pepper, and salt, and mix well. Form the shrimp mixture into patties, add 2 tablespoons of vegetable oil to a large sauté pan and cook over medium heat for 3-4 minutes per side. Reserve the cooked patties on a plate while you make the hollandaise sauce and poach the eggs.

Hollandaise sauce:
Melt the butter in a small saucepan. Meanwhile puree the egg yolks in a blender (if you do not have a blender you can make the hollandaise in a homemade double boiler; see below). With the blender running add the warm, melted butter in a slow stream. Add the lemon juice at the end.

To poach the eggs:
Bring 2 inches of water in a medium saucepan to a boil over high heat then turn the heat down to medium-low. Add 1 tablespoon of white vinegar. Gently crack an egg into a bowl then add the egg to the pan. Be careful not to break the yolk! We use prep bowls to slip the cracked egg slowly into the poaching liquid. Allow the egg to cook undisturbed for 3 minutes. Use a slotted spoon to remove the egg and gently place on top of the shrimp cake.

The final product:
Toast the English muffins, place a shrimp patty on each half of an English muffin, top with a poached egg and finish with a couple tablespoons of hollandaise over each muffin half.
Note: If you have the 2 cup sized food processor, you may have to puree the shrimp in a couple of batches.

Making hollandaise by hand:
Fill a saucepan with 2 inches of water and place on the stove over high heat and bring to a boil. Once the water is boiling reduce the heat to low. Whisk the egg yolks in a glass bowl and place the bowl on top of the saucepan. Make a homemade double boiler by placing the glass bowl over the saucepan. Whisk the egg yolks continuously until they become smooth and light yellow. While whisking, slowly drizzle the butter into the eggs. Once the sauce is thick you can turn off the heat and add the lemon juice.

MEMPHIS FRENCH TOAST SANDWICH

This is our twist on the king's signature sandwich.
It's the ultimate in comfort food for a lazy Saturday morning.

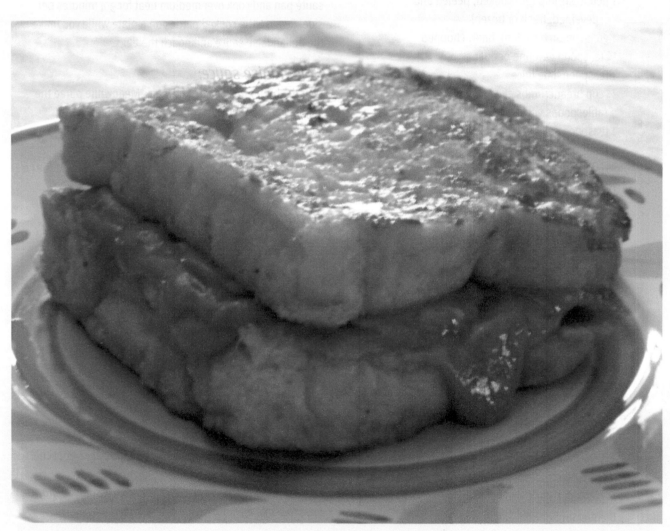

Servings: 6
Prep time: 10 minutes
Cook time: 4 minutes per batch
Cost: $8.18

Ingredients

12 pieces of bread, preferably Challah
2 bananas, thinly sliced
8 eggs
1 cup milk
12 tablespoons peanut butter (2 per sandwich)
6 tablespoons honey
4 tablespoons butter (1 tablespoon per batch)
¼ teaspoon ground nutmeg
Sugar for sprinkling

Equipment

Large sauté pan, preferably one that can fit 3 pieces
of bread
Mixing bowl x 2
Whisk
Measuring cups & spoons

Directions

1. Slice the bread into ½ inch thick slices.

2. Whisk the eggs, milk, and nutmeg in a bowl.

3. Heat a large sauté pan over medium heat.
   Melt 1 tablespoon of butter in the pan.
   Once the butter has melted, sprinkle about
   ½ teaspoon sugar over the melted butter.
   Dip each side of the bread in the egg mixture
   and place bread in the pan with the melted
   butter and sugar.
   Cook about 2 minutes per side.

4. In a separate, microwave-safe mixing bowl,
   mix together the honey and peanut butter
   and microwave for 60 seconds. Once you
   remove it, blend it thoroughly with a spoon.
   Slice 2 bananas directly into the honey peanut
   sauce and mix.
   Spread mixture over one half of a piece of French
   toast, cover with another piece of French toast
   and serve warm.

OMELET PROVENÇAL FOR ONE

This recipe gives you omelet know-how in a healthy, elegant template. We give you the ingredients of a typical French crepe without the added calorie count. Reuse the basic method and add your own ingredients to make whatever kind of omelet you want, whenever you want!

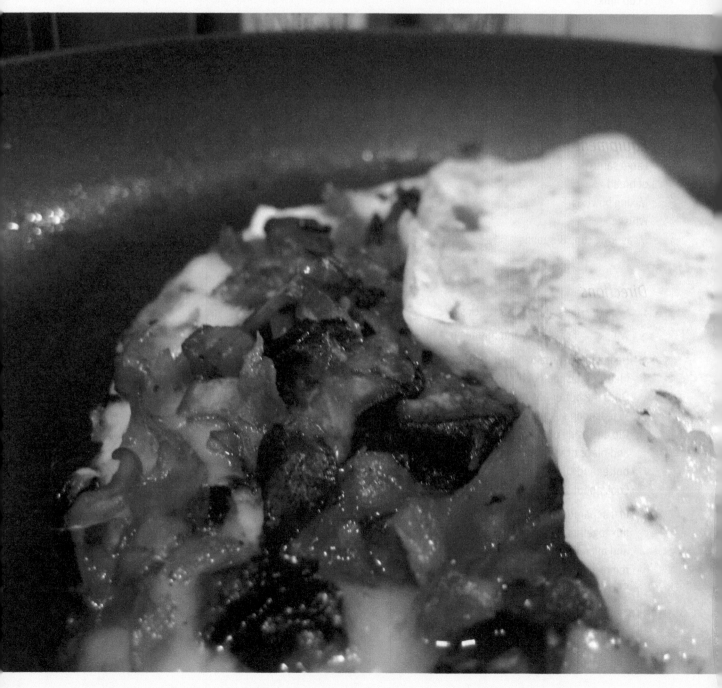

Servings: 1
Prep time: 15 minutes
Cooking time: 15 minutes
Cost: $11.38

Ingredients

4 large fresh eggs (whites only)
1 tablespoon milk (or half and half)
1 ½ cups Swiss cheese, shredded
¼ teaspoon black pepper
½ teaspoon salt
1 small shallot, minced
¼ teaspoon sugar
3 slices deli ham, chiffonade
    (cut in thin, ribbon-like strips)
1 cup portabella mushrooms,
    sliced into thinly
½ teaspoon rosemary leaves
½ teaspoon chives
¼ teaspoon thyme
4 tablespoons unsalted butter

Equipment

Large sauté/frying pan
Spatula & Whisk
Mixing bowl
Chopping knife
Measuring cups & spoons

Directions

1. Melt the first tablespoon of butter in a pan over low heat. Butter burns easily, so be sure not to get it going until you're ready to start.
   Once the butter has melted and covered the surface of the entire pan, add the minced shallot, portabella mushrooms, and ham.
   Sprinkle the sugar over the ham as it's cooking and add in the chives and thyme, stirring occasionally to mix the flavors of the herbs with the juice from the ham, mushrooms, and shallots. Season with salt and pepper.
   Allow to simmer on medium-low heat for about 10 minutes.

2. In the meantime, break the eggs and remove the yolk, pouring the egg whites into a mixing bowl.
   You may want to keep a separate container to store the leftover yolk for a quick snack later.
   Add the rosemary and milk to the mixture. Whisk thoroughly.

3. Next, move the cooked ingredients to a separate dish. Using the same pan, melt another 2 tablespoons of butter over low heat and slowly pour in the egg mixture. An omelet can burn very quickly if there isn't enough butter (or olive oil alternatively) on the pan, so don't be stingy!
   Sprinkle the side facing you with the Swiss cheese. Cook for about 2 minutes.
   To check the bottom of the omelet, gently left from the edge of the pan with a spatula once the egg whites have begun to solidify.

4. Add the ham, mushrooms, and onions back into the omelet, covering half the egg.
   Cook for about 1 minute, then fold the other side of the egg over very delicately using the spatula.
   Cook for another 1 – 2 minutes, until the middle has cooked through.
   Gingerly remove the omelet and enjoy!

BAJA BREAKFAST BONANZA

Wake up with a kick! This spicy breakfast sizzler will blast you off your seat and deliver a whopping punch of protein to get you through your busy day. Saddle up your horse, because the juicy chorizo meat and tender cactus flavors are sure to transport you to the fiery Wild West. It's a meal in a wrap!

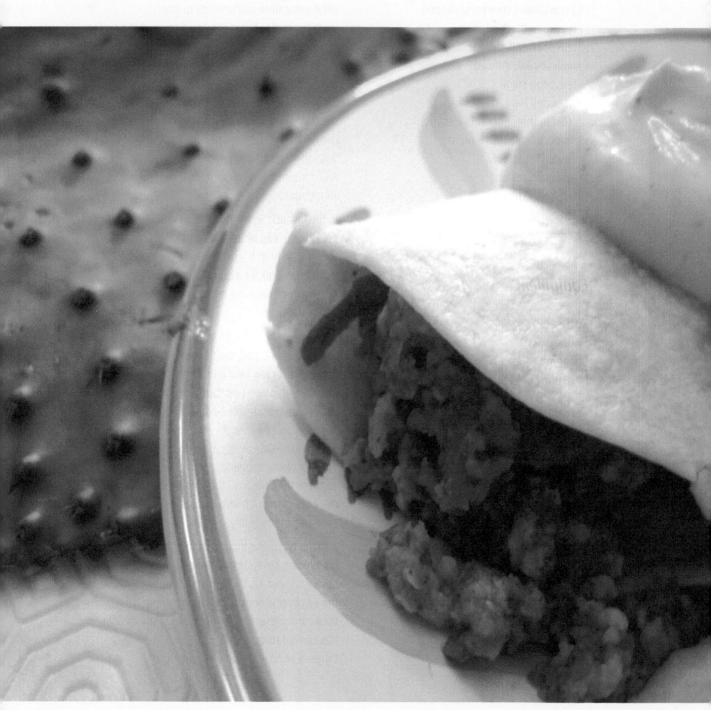

Servings: 6
Prep time: 10 minutes
Cooking time: 20 minutes
Cost: $16.33

Ingredients

1 lb. chorizo meat (found in the sausage area
    or in the chilled Mexican area)
8 oz. tender cactus meat (available in most
    supermarkets in the Mexican aisle)
6 large fresh eggs
1 ½ cups shredded Monterey Jack or Colby Jack
cheese
6 squirts hot sauce
1/8 teaspoon ground cinnamon
½ teaspoon salt
1/8 teaspoon black pepper
1 tablespoon onion powder
¼ cup chopped fresh cilantro
2 tablespoons olive oil
6 soft tortillas
1 tablespoon skim milk or low fat milk
    or half and half
1 x 12 oz. can tomatillos
1 tablespoon lime juice
Chili Lime Sour Cream (see below)

Chili Lime Sour Cream

1 cup sour cream
1/8 teaspoon cayenne pepper
2 tablespoons lime juice

Equipment

Large sauté pan
Chopping knife
Cutting board
Whisk
Large & small mixing bowls
Measuring cups & spoons
Spatula or wooden spoon

Directions

1. In a mixing bowl, combine the egg and milk, whisking thoroughly. Set aside. Dice the tomatillos and drizzle with 1 tablespoon of lime juice. Set this aside as well.

2. Set the stove to medium heat and lightly drizzle a large sauté pan with 1 tablespoon of olive oil. Once the pan is warm, place the tortilla shells one by one in the pan and allow to warm for one minute on each side. Remove and set aside.

3. Using the same large sauté pan, heat another tablespoon of olive oil over medium-low. Chop up the chorizo meat into tiny chunks, making sure you have removed the thin, sheer outer casing, and place directly onto the warmed pan. Sprinkle with the hot sauce, salt, onion powder, and cinnamon, making sure that the flavoring goes directly on the meat.
Allow to heat at the same temperature for about 8 – 10 minutes.
Drain the cactus meat and add it to the warmed chorizo mixture

4. While the meat is cooking, you can combine the sour cream, cayenne pepper, and lime juice.
Mix thoroughly with a spoon in a small bowl.

5. Add the chopped cilantro to the meat and stir.
Now, you're ready for the eggs.
Slowly pour the egg mixture from the mixing bowl onto the meat.
Do not stir! After about 2 minutes, add the cheese. Cook for another 1 – 2 minutes (until the cheese has melted).

6. Spoon a generous portion of the mix onto each tortilla and fold over.
Top with the sour cream and tomatillos and serve for a zesty morning meal.

12. Ice Cream Factory

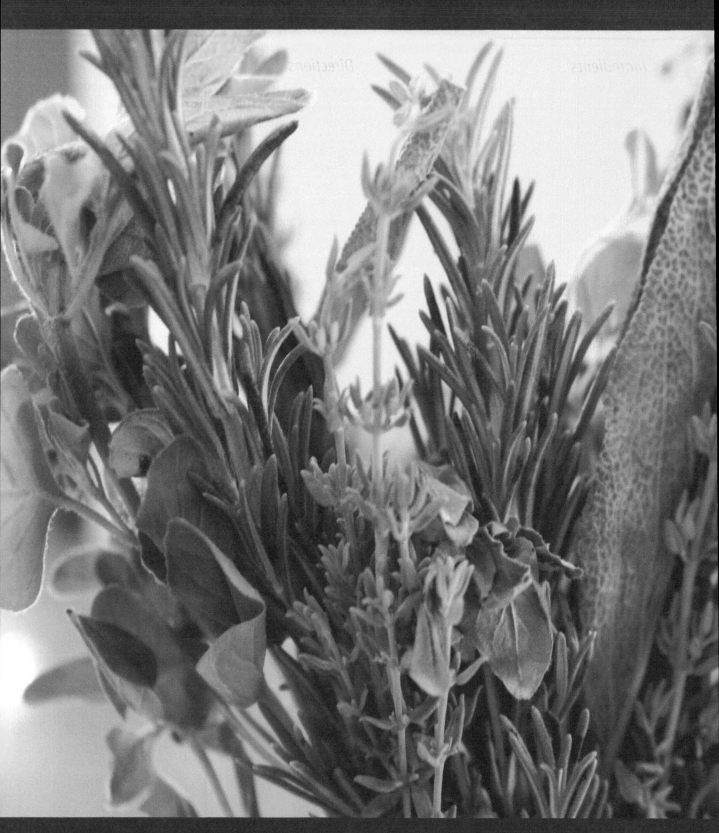

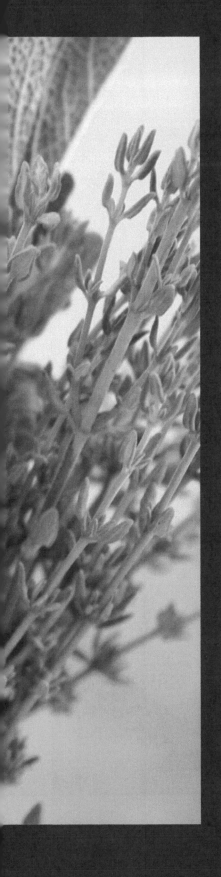

Lavender Ice Cream Sandwiches

Pink Peppercorn Ice Cream

Saffron Ice Cream

Pakistani Cardamom Almond Ice Cream

Thyme Ice Cream

Cilantro Ice Cream with Chocolate-Corn Cake

New Orleans Chocolate Cayenne
Ice Cream Sandwiches

Captain Crunch Ice Cream

LAVENDER ICE CREAM SANDWICHES

The French have been using lavender in cooking for hundreds of years. Lavender adds a sweet, delicate flavor to foods. We've paired this floral ice cream with a chocolaty cookie making an elegant flavor combination that can't be beat.

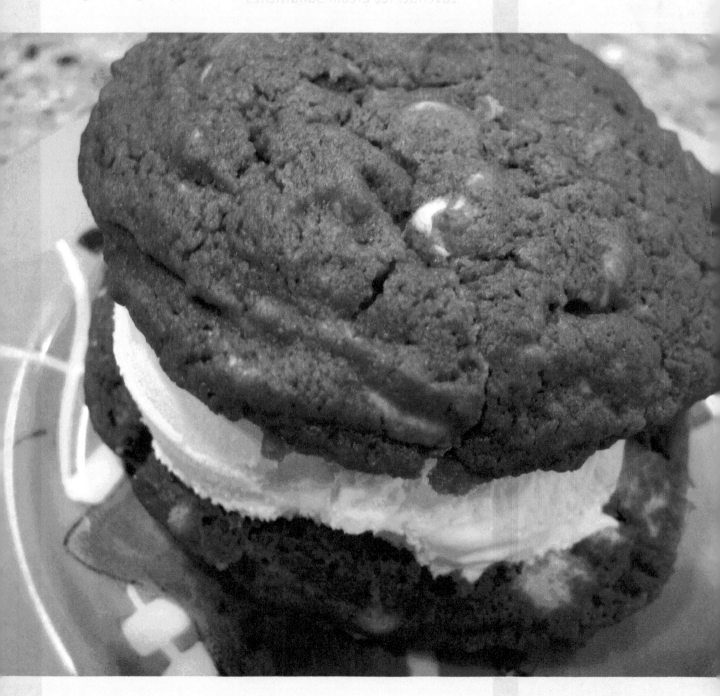

Servings: 5 - 6
Prep time: 15 minutes
Cooking time: 30 minutes
Cost: $9.57

Ingredients

Ice Cream
2 cups heavy cream
1 cup milk
4 egg yolks
½ cup sugar
2 tablespoons lavender (dried buds)

Cookies
17.5 oz. sugar cookie mix
½ cup unsweetened cocoa powder
1 cup white chocolate chips
1 stick unsalted butter + 4 tablespoons
2 eggs

Equipment
1 quart ice cream maker
Homemade double boiler (saucepan + glass bowl)
1 ½ - 2 quart saucepan
Whisk and wooden spoon
Baking sheets
Ice cream scoop
Mixing bowl & measuring cups
Strainer

Directions

For the ice cream:
1. Pour the milk, cream, and sugar into a saucepan over medium-low heat until the sugar dissolves; add lavender and heat slowly for about 5-8 minutes to infuse the liquid with lavender.
2. Strain the lavender-cream mixture to remove the lavender.
3. In a glass bowl whisk the egg yolks.
4. Meanwhile, make a homemade double boiler: take a 2 quart sauce pan, add 2 inches of water and place over medium-high heat until the water boils, then reduce the heat to low.
   Next, place the glass bowl with the eggs over the saucepan.
5. Slowly add the lavender-cream to the eggs while whisking continuously. Cook over low heat until the custard coats the back of a wooden spoon—this will take about 5-8 minutes.
6. Place the custard in the refrigerator for a couple of hours or overnight.

For the cookies:
1. Preheat the oven to 375 degrees F.
2. Combine the cookie mix, cocoa, and chocolate chips until well blended. Soften the butter in the microwave for 15 seconds or leave on the counter for a couple of hours. Add the butter and eggs to the dry ingredients and mix until dough forms.
   Use your ice cream scoop to make large cookies.
   This batter should make 11-12 large cookies.
   Bake for 14 to 16 minutes.
3. You should keep the bowl and beater of your ice cream maker in the freezer.
   After 2 hours, pour the custard into the ice cream maker bowl (it will be liquid at this stage) and run the machine according to the manufacturer's instructions.
   Transfer to a freezer-safe container and store in the freezer.
4. You'll have to wait for the cookies to cool and the ice cream to harden before assembling the sandwiches.
   It's best to do this just before serving.

PINK PEPPERCORN ICE CREAM

This is sweet and so interesting. It's an elegant end to any meal— or an elegant midnight snack!

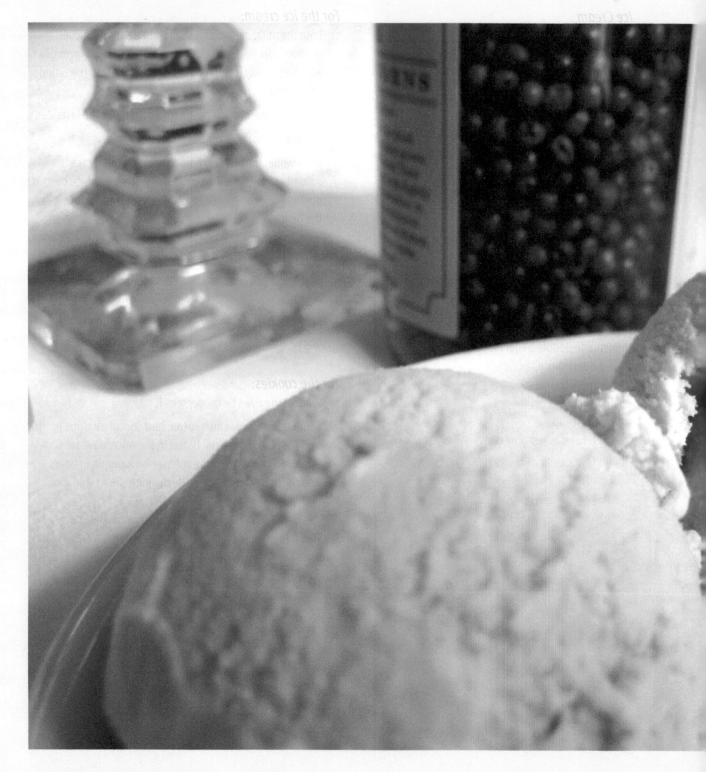

Servings: 6 - 8
Prep time: 5 minutes
Cooking time: 15 minutes
Cost: $3.00

Ingredients
2 cups heavy cream
1 cup milk
4 egg yolks
½ cup sugar
½ teaspoon pink peppercorns (ground)
3 drops red food coloring

Equipment
Peppermill or spice grinder
1-quart ice cream maker
Homemade double boiler—glass bowl and sauce pan
1 ½ to 2-quart saucepan
Whisk and wooden spoon
Measuring cups & spoons

Directions
1. Heat the milk, cream, and sugar over medium-low heat until the sugar has dissolved.
   Add the ground peppercorns once the sugar has dissolved and cook for 5-8 minutes. This will allow the sugar to melt and to infuse the cream mixture with peppercorn flavor.

2. Whisk the egg yolks in a glass mixing bowl.

3. Meanwhile, make a homemade double boiler:
   take a 2 quart sauce pan, add 2 inches of water and place over medium-high heat until the water boils, then reduce the heat to low.
   Next, place the glass bowl with the eggs over the saucepan.
   Slowly add the peppercorn-cream to the eggs while whisking continuously—it is very important to add the hot cream slowly. This process is called tempering (bringing the eggs up to the same temperature as a hot liquid in order not to scramble them).

4. Cook over low heat until the mixture coats the back of a wooden spoon. This will take about 5-8 minutes. You've now made a custard.

5. Put the custard in the refrigerator for 2-3 hours or over night.

6. Once your custard has cooled, add the food coloring and mix, then put it in the ice cream maker and churn until it is almost solid.
   This takes about 30 minutes. You can serve directly out of the ice cream maker or freeze it for an hour before serving.

Secret tip: use a coffee grinder to grind your spices. You can purchase these for about $20. They are great to have around to freshly grind spices for Indian cooking.

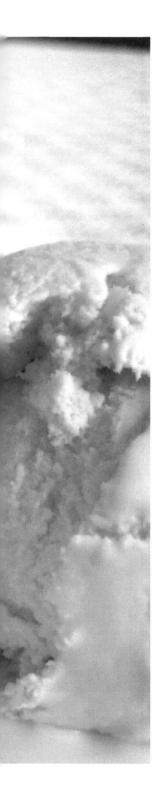

SAFFRON
ICE CREAM

Saffron may be the most expensive spice in the world, but once you've tasted this ice cream you won't care! It's perhaps the most incredible taste experience you will ever have. Try it with apple pie; it goes wonderfully with French tarte tartin (French apple pie). Ellen's husband created this years before it appeared in gelato bars.

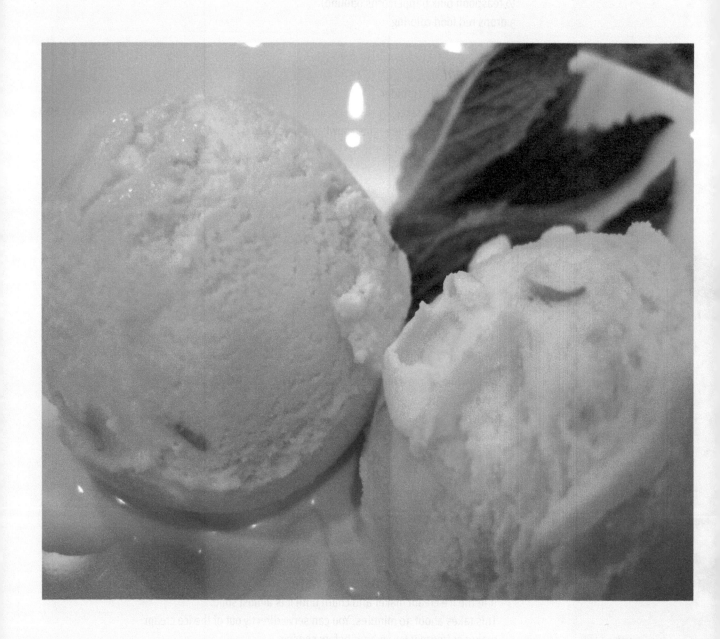

Servings: 6 - 8
Prep time: 5 minutes
Cooking time: 15 minutes
Cost: $5.11

Ingredients

2 cups heavy cream
1 cups milk
4 egg yolks
½ cup sugar
1 teaspoon saffron threads

Equipment

1 quart ice cream maker
Homemade double boiler—glass bowl and sauce pan
1 ½ to 2 quart sauce pan
Whisk and wooden spoon
Measuring cups & spoons

Directions

1. Heat the milk, cream, sugar, and saffron over medium-low heat until the sugar has dissolved and the saffron has infused the mixture. This takes about 5-8 minutes. The mixture will appear yellow from the saffron. Don't worry if all the saffron threads do not melt—they'll look beautiful in the finished ice cream.

2. Whisk the egg yolks in a glass bowl.
    Meanwhile, make a homemade double boiler: take a 2 quart sauce pan, add 2 inches of water and place over medium-high heat until the water boils, then reduce the heat to low.
    Next, place the glass bowl with the eggs over the saucepan. Slowly add the saffron-milk to the eggs while whisking continuously.
    Cook over low heat until the custard coats the back of a wooden spoon; this will take about 5-8 minutes.

3. Put custard in the refrigerator for 2-3 hours or overnight.

4. Put the ice cream in your ice cream maker and churn until it is almost solid. This takes about 30 minutes. You can serve it just out of the ice cream maker or put it in the freezer for an hour or two, to solidify further.

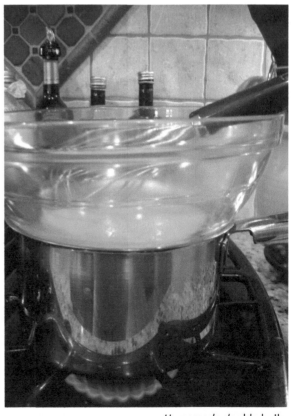

Homemade double boiler

PAKISTANI CARDAMOM ALMOND ICE CREAM

For a mouthful of the authentic world of exotic Pakistani desserts, sit back and buckle up for a direct flight to the other side of the globe. We've recreated a classic pudding-like dish that traditionally cools and firms up in individually sized terra cotta bowls. This will really hit the spot on a hot summer night. The burst of cardamom flavor is like opening the door to a pantry in Lahore, and the crunch of the almond slivers adds a level of texture that, in this dish, sure beats the old standby of chocolate chips! A little gift from Sophia's childhood to your kitchen.

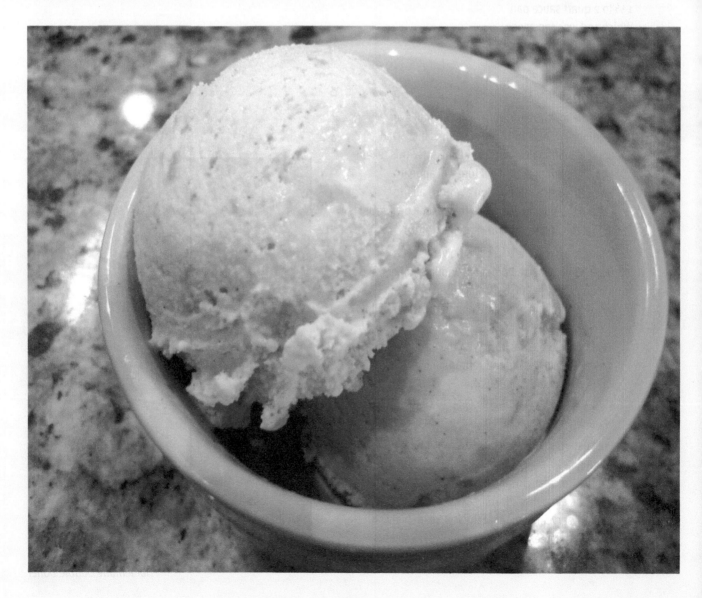

Servings: 6 - 8
Prep time: 5 minutes
Cooking time: 15 minutes
Cost: $4.75

Ingredients
2 cups heavy cream
1 cup milk
½ cup sugar
4 egg yolks
2 teaspoons ground cardamom
2 oz. package blanched slivered almonds

Equipment
1-quart ice cream maker
Homemade double boiler—glass bowl and sauce pan
1 ½ to 2-quart sauce pan
Whisk and wooden spoon
Measuring cups & spoons

Directions
1. Pour the milk, cream, sugar, and cardamom into a saucepan over medium-low heat; warm for 5 to 8 minutes, until the sugar has dissolved, mixing occasionally.

2. Whisk the egg yolks in a glass bowl.
   Meanwhile, make a homemade double boiler: take a 2 quart sauce pan, add 2 inches of water and place over medium-high heat until the water boils then reduce the heat to low. Next, place the glass bowl with the eggs over the saucepan. Ladle the warm cream mixture into the eggs slowly in order to temper the eggs. Whisk continuously during this process. (Tempering slowly brings up the temperature of an egg mixture so that the eggs don't scramble.)

3. Cook over low heat until the custard coats the back of a wooden spoon. This will take about 5-8 minutes.

4. Cool the custard in the refrigerator for 2-3 hours or overnight. Once the custard has cooled add it to your ice cream maker, add the almonds, and churn for 30 minutes.
   This can be eaten directly out of the ice cream maker for a softer version. Transfer to a freezer-safe container and store in the freezer for a firmer version.

THYME
ICE CREAM

Savory ice creams are the latest craze. We think this craze is here to stay!

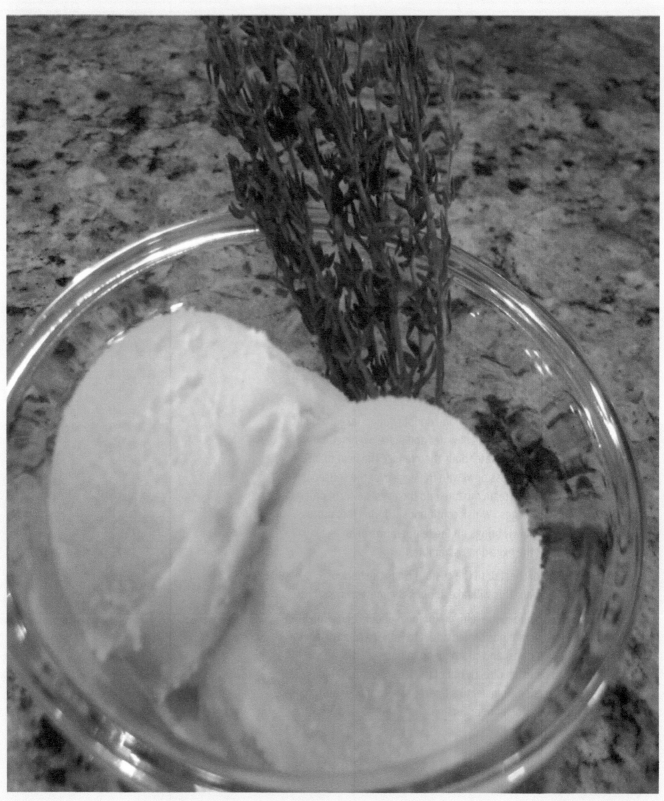

Servings: 4 - 6
Prep time: 15 minutes
Cooking time: 15 minutes
Cost: $2.27

Ingredients

1 cup of milk
2 cups of heavy cream
4 egg yolks
½ cup sugar
¼ teaspoon ground thyme or 8 sprigs fresh thyme

Equipment

1-quart ice cream maker
Homemade double boiler—glass bowl and sauce pan
1 ½ to 2-quart sauce pan
Whisk
Wooden spoon

Directions

1. Pour the milk, cream, sugar, and ground thyme (or the sprigs) into a saucepan over medium-low heat; warm for 5 to 8 minutes.

2. Whisk the egg yolks in a glass bowl.

3. Meanwhile, make a homemade double boiler: take a 2 quart sauce pan, add 2 inches of water and place over medium-high heat until the water boils then reduce the heat to low.
   Next, place the glass bowl with the eggs over the saucepan. Ladle the warm cream mixture into the eggs slowly in order to temper the eggs.
   Whisk continuously during this process. (Tempering slowly brings up the temperature of an egg mixture so that the eggs don't scramble.)

4. Cook over low heat until the custard coats the back of a wooden spoon. This will take about 5 to 8 minutes.

5. Put custard in the refrigerator for 2-3 hours or overnight. Once the custard has cooled add it to your ice cream maker and churn for 30 minutes. This can be eaten directly out of the ice cream maker for a softer version.
   Transfer to a freezer-safe container and store in the freezer for a firmer version.

CILANTRO ICE CREAM WITH CHOCOLATE-CORN CAKE

This unusual dessert will wow your guests. It may seem like a strange flavor for an ice cream, but it's really a vibrant and bright flavor! When paired with the chocolate-corn cake, you'll feel like you're in a 5-star restaurant in Acapulco.

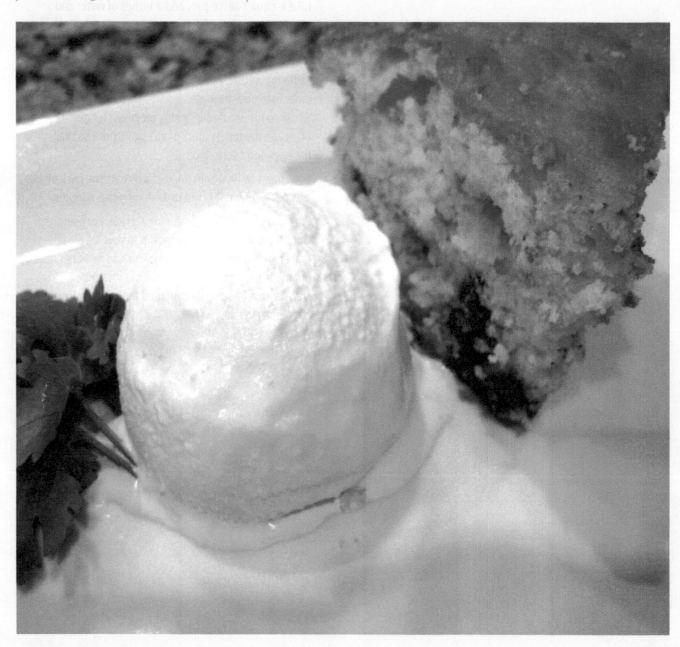

Servings: 6 - 8
Prep time: 10 minutes
Cooking time: 1 hour
Cost: $10.42

Ingredients

Ice cream

2 cups heavy cream
1 cup milk
4 egg yolks
½ cup sugar
1 cup fresh cilantro leaves, rinsed

Chocolate-Corn Cake

18 oz. box of yellow cake mix
8.5 oz. box of corn muffin mix
4 eggs
1 ¾ cups milk
1 cup chocolate chips
1 cup canned sweet corn
1 stick unsalted butter, melted
2 tablespoons flour
Pinch of kosher salt
Pinch of ground black pepper (optional)

Equipment

Large mixing bowl
9 x 13 inch baking dish
Hand mixer (optional) *
1-quart ice cream maker
Homemade double boiler
    (glass bowl and saucepan)
1 ½ - 2-quart saucepan
Whisk and wooden spoon

Directions

1. Heat the milk, cream, and sugar over medium-low heat until the sugar has dissolved (2-3 minutes).
Add the cilantro and cook for 15 minutes over medium-low heat. This will allow the cilantro to infuse the cream. Strain the mixture to remove the cilantro leaves.

2. Whisk the egg yolks in a glass bowl.

3. Meanwhile, make a homemade double boiler:
take a 2 quart sauce pan, add 2 inches of water and place over medium-high heat until the water boils then reduce the heat to low. Next, place the glass bowl with the eggs over the saucepan. Slowly add the cilantro-cream to the eggs while whisking continuously.
Cook until the custard coats the back of a wooden spoon. This will take about 5-8 minutes.

4. Put custard in the refrigerator for 2-3 hours or overnight.

5. Pour the custard into your ice cream maker and churn until it is almost solid. This takes about 30 minutes. You can serve it directly out of the ice cream maker or put it in the freezer for an hour or two for a firmer consistency.

For the cake:

1. Preheat the oven to 350 degrees F.

2. Mix together the cake mixes, eggs, butter, and milk until smooth. (Add a dash of ground black pepper if you want a spicy kick.) If you are not using a hand mixer, melt the butter in the microwave for 30 seconds and use a whisk to mix the batter—it may take 3 to 4 minutes of mixing to get a smooth batter.

3. Mix the chocolate chips and corn with the flour—this will prevent them from sinking to the bottom of the cake.

4. Add the chocolate chips and corn and pour into a greased 9x13 inch-baking dish. Bake for 45 minutes.

5. Cool for 15-20 minutes before serving.

6. Serve the cake with the ice cream after a southwestern or Mexican dinner.

Hand mixers cost about $20 and are well worth the investment!

NEW ORLEANS CHOCOLATE CAYENNE ICE CREAM SANDWICHES

Spicy cayenne pepper in ice cream? Absolutely! Remember the rule for spicy foods: your best option for counteracting the spice is with dairy products. This ice cream is not as spicy as it sounds. Actually the cayenne adds an interesting twist—quiz your friends on the secret ingredient. They'll never guess it is cayenne pepper.

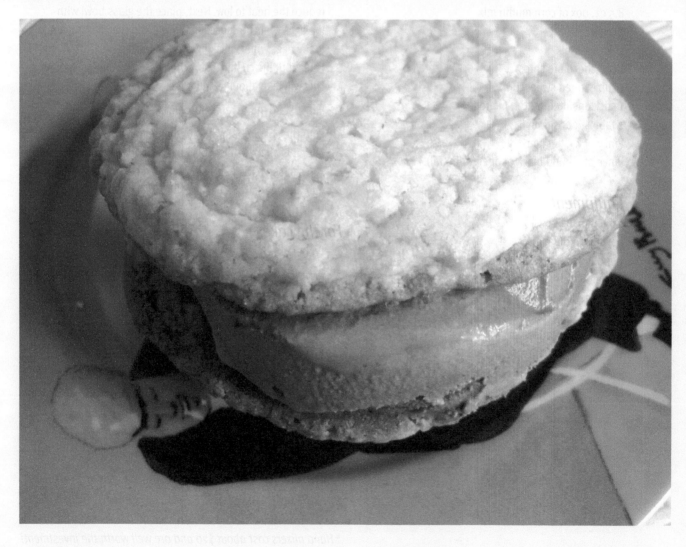

Servings: 5 – 6
Prep time: 15 minutes
Cooking time: 30 minutes
Cost: $8.05

Ingredients
Ice Cream
2 cups heavy cream
1 cup milk
½ cup sugar
½ cup unsweetened cocoa powder
4 egg yolks
¼ teaspoon cayenne pepper

Cookies
17.5 oz. package of sugar cookie mix
1 teaspoon orange zest
2 teaspoons almond extract
1 egg
1 stick unsalted butter, softened
(you can microwave for 15 seconds in wrapper)

Equipment
1-quart ice cream maker
Homemade double boiler
   (glass bowl and sauce pan)
1 ½ to 2-quart sauce pan
Whisk
Wooden spoon
Soup ladle
Baking sheet
Large ice cream scoop
Measuring cups & spoons

Directions
Note: You should keep the bowl and beater of your ice cream maker in the freezer so you are always ready to make homemade ice cream.

For the ice cream:
1. Pour the milk, cream, vanilla, sugar, cocoa, and cayenne pepper into a saucepan over medium-low heat; warm for 5 to 8 minutes.

2. Whisk the egg yolks in a glass bowl.

3. Meanwhile, make a homemade double boiler: take a 2 quart sauce pan, add 2 inches of water and place over medium-high heat until the water boils then reduce the heat to low. Next, place the glass bowl with the eggs over the saucepan. Ladle the warm cream mixture into the eggs slowly in order to temper the eggs. Whisk continuously during this process. (Tempering slowly brings up the temperature of an egg mixture so that the eggs don't scramble.)

4. Cook over low heat until the custard coats the back of a wooden spoon. This will take about 5-8 minutes.

5. Put custard in the refrigerator for 2-3 hours or overnight. Once the custard has cooled add it to your ice cream maker and churn for 30 minutes. This can be eaten directly out of the ice cream maker for a softer version. Transfer to a freezer-safe container and store in the freezer for a traditional ice cream texture.

For the cookies:
1. Preheat the oven to 350 degrees F.

2. Mix together all the cookies ingredients until you have a soft dough. Use your large ice cream scoop to drop the balls of dough onto the cookie sheet.

3. Bake for 14 minutes. Let cool and make these delicious sandwiches.

CAPTAIN CRUNCH ICE CREAM

This is breakfast for dessert! We've used egg whites instead of yolks for a velvety texture.
You can use the base for many different ice creams—you can add anything your heart desires—
chocolate chips, fruit, candy, etc.

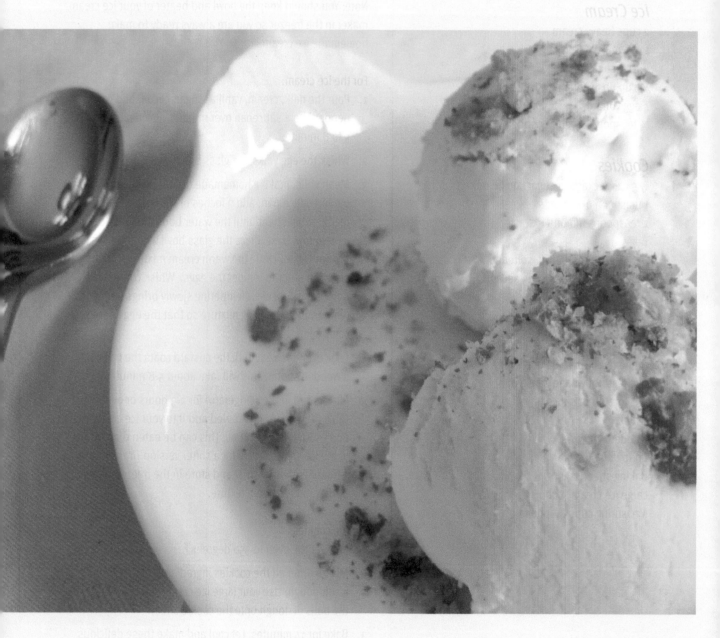

Servings: 6-8
Prep time: 5 minutes
Cooking time: 15 minutes
Cost: $ 4.26

Ingredients

2 cups heavy cream
1 cup milk
½ cup sugar
2 teaspoons vanilla
4 egg whites
1 cup Captain Crunch's Crunch Berries cereal
+ extra for sprinkling

Equipment

Homemade double boiler (sauce pan + glass bowl)
2-quart sauce pan
Whisk
Wooden spoon
1-quart ice cream maker

Directions

1. Put the heavy cream, milk, and sugar in a 2-quart saucepan and heat over medium-high heat until it comes to a simmer (small bubbles on the edge of the pan). Turn the heat off.

2. Put about 2 inches of water in another sauce pan and heat over medium-high heat until it comes to a slow boil—turn the heat down to medium low. This is the base of your homemade double boiler—see the recipe for Saffron Ice Cream for a picture of the double boiler. Place the egg whites in your glass bowl and add about ½ cup of the warm cream to temper the eggs (tempering means bringing the egg mixture up to the same temperature as the warm cream slowly so not to scramble the eggs). Whisk constantly during this process.

3. Add another ½ cup of warm milk then add entire cream mixture to the eggs (using a soup ladle for this makes it easier). Place the glass bowl over the simmering water and cook over medium-low heat until the custard coats the back of a wooden spoon—this takes about 5-8 minutes.

4. Cool the custard in the refrigerator for about 2 to 3 hours. Place in your ice cream maker. It will take about 30 minutes for the ice cream to form.

5. Add the Captain Crunch cereal once the ice cream has been churning for about 20 minutes.

6. Crumble cereal over your ice cream before serving. The sweet crunch is wonderful.

13. MAKE YOUR OWN GOURMET PIZZA

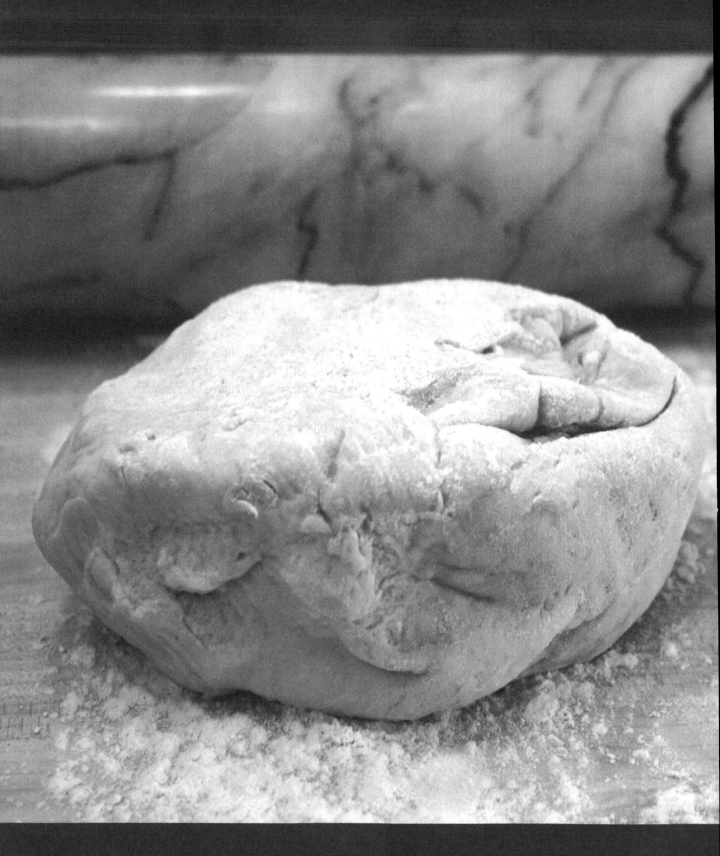

Pizza Bella

Shrimp Caesar Salad Pizza

New Orleans Crab Béchamel Pizza

Antipasto Pizza

Nutella Pizza

Smoked Salmon Pizza

Pesto Pizza

Tuna Artichoke Pizza

Make Your Own Pizza Party

PIZZA BELLA

A twist on our fig and Gorgonzola bites, this gourmet pizza is easy and fun to put together at a big gathering. Minimum prep and cooking time add to its appeal for large crowds.

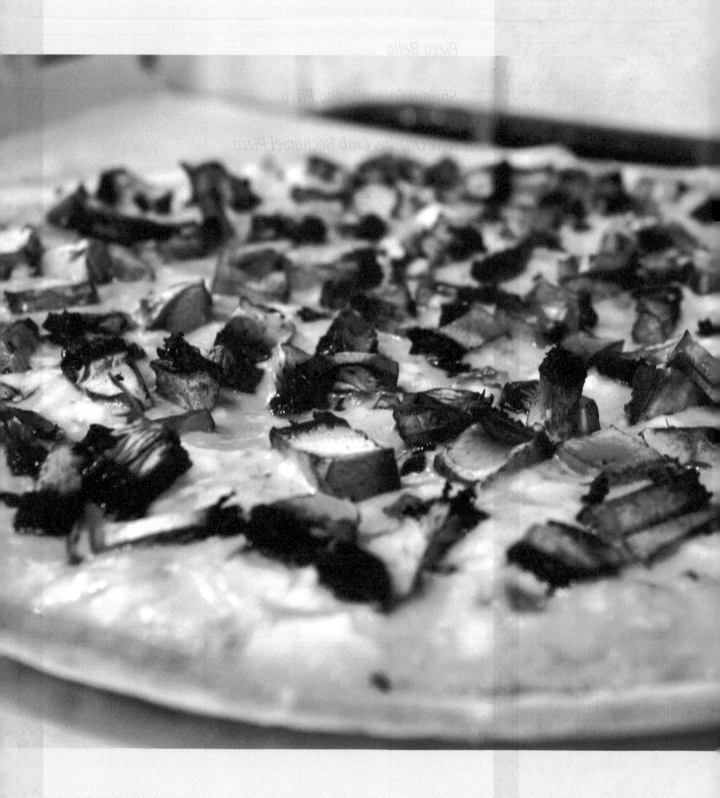

Servings: 4 – 6
Prep time: 5 minutes
Cooking time: 8 ½ minutes
Cost: $10.90

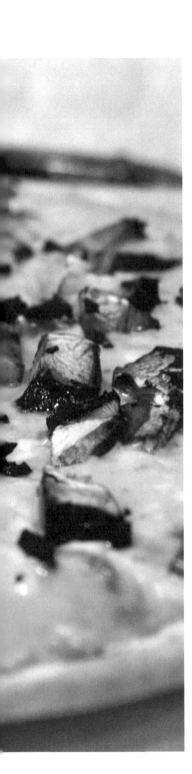

Ingredients
1 plain pre-made 12" thin crust pizza
8 oz. Gorgonzola
2 heaping tablespoons of fig spread
2 oz. portabella mushrooms, thinly sliced
2 tablespoons of olive oil

Equipment
Microwave-safe bowl
Paring knife
Spreading knife (a cake knife works great here)
Cookie sheet (optional)

Directions
1. Preheat the oven to 425 degrees F.

2. Remove the Gorgonzola from the package and microwave for 45 seconds (until soft).

3. Mix the fig spread with the Gorgonzola until the Gorgonzola takes on a spreadable consistency. Spread the Gorgonzola-fig mix over the pizza crust. Do NOT put any olive oil on the pizza itself just yet!

4. After spreading the Gorgonzola and fig sauce over the pizza crust sprinkle with sliced mushroom, distributing them evenly.
   Now you can drizzle the olive oil evenly over the pizza.

5. Place either on a cookie sheet or directly onto the oven rack for 8 ½ minutes or until the Gorgonzola first begins to bubble. Remove and serve.

SHRIMP CAESAR SALAD PIZZA

The crunch of fresh lettuce leaves on this salad is wonderful. For an authentic Caesar touch, throw a couple of anchovies on top.

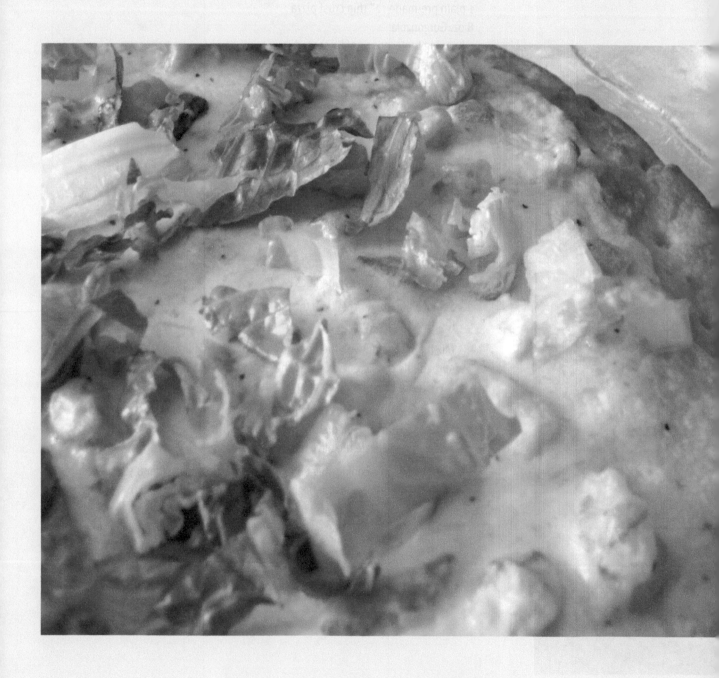

Servings: 4 – 6
Prep time: 10 minutes
Cooking time: 10 minutes
Cost: $6.61

Ingredients

½ cup ricotta cheese
½ cup Caesar dressing
¼ cup grated or shredded parmesan
½ cup shredded romaine lettuce
¼ cup lemon juice
1 cup chopped, cooked shrimp (about ½ pound)
1 pre-made thin pizza crust

Equipment

Baking sheet (optional, you can put the crust directly
on the oven rack)
Mixing bowls
Measuring cups & spoons

Directions

1. Prepare the pizza crust according to package
   directions.

2. Marinate the pre-cooked, chopped shrimp in
   lemon juice in a mixing bowl for about 5 minutes.

3. While the shrimp soaks in the lemon juice,
   mix the ricotta and Caesar dressing thoroughly
   in a small bowl and then spread over the pizza
   crust.

4. Distribute the pieces of shrimp over the ricotta-
   Caesar mixture, then sprinkle with Parmesan.

5. Bake for 8 – 10 minutes according to package
   directions.

6. Once you have removed the pizza, spread
   shredded romaine over the top and sprinkle
   with lemon juice and more Parmesan for a fresh,
   crispy taste.

NEW ORLEANS CRAB BÉCHAMEL PIZZA

Sure to be a favorite pizza to those with a taste for seafood, we simultaneously teach you how to make a béchamel sauce and classy pizza in one simple recipe.

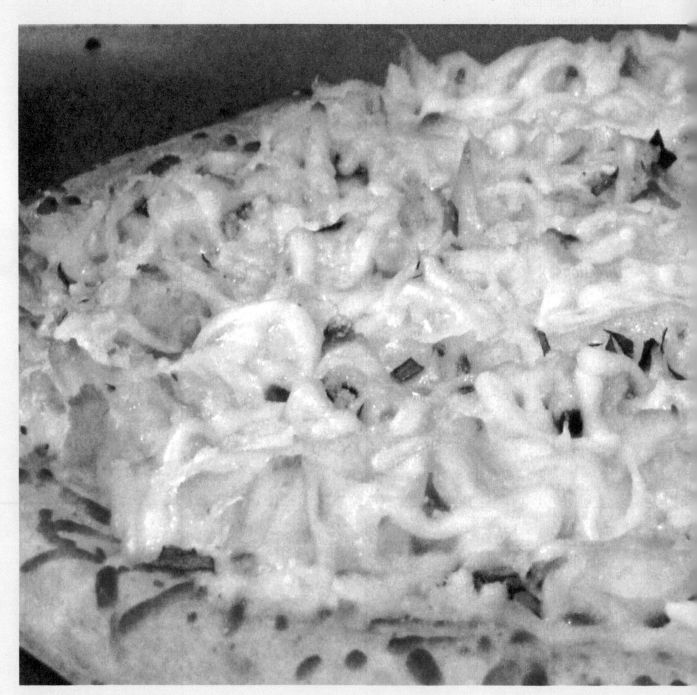

Servings: 4
Prep time: 10 minutes
Cooking time: 20 minutes
Cost: $9.39

Ingredients

1 plain pre-made 12" thin pizza crust
Béchamel sauce (see below)
8 oz. crab meat
2 tablespoons chopped tarragon
1 cup shredded mozzarella cheese
2 tablespoons grated Parmesan cheese

Béchamel Sauce Ingredients

(enough for 2 pizzas)
2 tablespoons unsalted butter
2 tablespoons all-purpose flour
2 cups of whole milk
½ cup diced sweet onion
    (half of a medium size onion)
½ teaspoon salt
¼ teaspoon black pepper
¼ teaspoon ground nutmeg

Equipment

Saucepan
Baking sheet (for a crispier crust, place pizza
    directly on oven rack)
Whisk or wooden spoon
Measuring cups and spoons

Directions

Preheat the oven according to the pizza crust package directions.

To make the béchamel sauce:

1. In a saucepan, melt 2 tablespoons of butter over medium-low heat. Add the onion and cook for 5 minutes.

2. Add the flour and cook for about one minute (until the mixture is light tan in color). Add nutmeg, salt, and pepper to the pan and stir.

3. Slowly add milk to the pan, stirring constantly to avoid creating a lumpy texture. Bring to a boil over medium-high heat, then reduce the heat and cook over medium-low for approximately 8-10 minutes, until thick. Stir occasionally as it thickens. (Many experts recommend adding heated milk to make a béchamel sauce to reduce the chance of having a lumpy mixture—we have found that cold milk works as long as you add it slowly and stir constantly.)

4. On a cutting board, chop two tablespoons of tarragon leaves finely (be sure to remove the leaves from the woody stems).

5. Top the pizza crust with béchamel sauce, crab, tarragon, and cheese and bake for 8-10 minutes.

*You can use the leftover Béchamel sauce to make a Mornay sauce. Traditional Mornay sauce is made with Gruyère cheese. We recommend making a "student's Mornay" by adding ¼ cup of any cheese you have in the refrigerator, warm over low heat, and serve over an omelet the next morning or over a white fish or shrimp for dinner.

ANTIPASTO PIZZA

We've brought the classic Italian appetizer of melon and prosciutto to an American pizza slice in this refreshing fusion recipe. It's an ultimate battle of salty and sweet with the tender proscuitto and juicy melon, balanced out by the light white cheeses serving as the base of this innovative white pie. Who says you can't have appetizers for dinner?

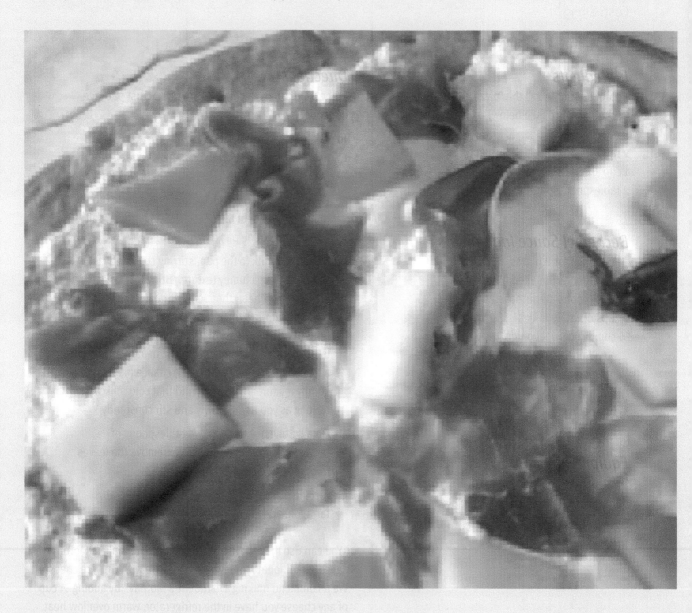

Servings: 4 – 6
Prep time: 10 minutes
Cooking time: 10 minutes
Cost: $13.48

Ingredients
1 cup fresh cantaloupe melon, thinly sliced
1 cup fresh honeydew melon, thinly sliced
1 cup ricotta cheese
¼ teaspoon salt
1/8 teaspoon black pepper
¼ cup grated Parmesan
1 ball fresh mozzarella cheese
½ pound prosciutto (Italian ham, found in the deli section
    of the market)
1 thin crust prepared pizza crust

Equipment
Measuring cups & spoons
Baking sheet (optional; you can put the pizza directly
    on the oven rack)
Paring knife
Mixing bowl

Directions
1. Prepare pizza crust according to package directions.

2. In a small mixing bowl, combine the ricotta, salt, and pepper.
   Spread the ricotta over the crust.

3. Slice the fresh mozzarella into thick slices and distribute evenly
   over the ricotta layer.

4. Sprinkle with the parmesan and pop into the oven (either
   directly onto the rack or on a baking dish) for about 8 – 10
   minutes, until the mozzarella chunks have begun to melt
   and the crust has browned.

5. While the pizza is baking, cut the melon into slices thin
   enough to fit into your mouth. Separate the prosciutto into
   small strips; you can easily do it by hand.

6. After the pizza has finished baking, place the melon on top
   of the melted cheese. Fill the spaces in between melon chunks
   with prosciutto, cut, and serve.

NUTELLA PIZZA

*Yes, we love chocolate hazelnut spread. We'll use it in almost anything.
This dessert pizza will end any meal with pizzazz.*

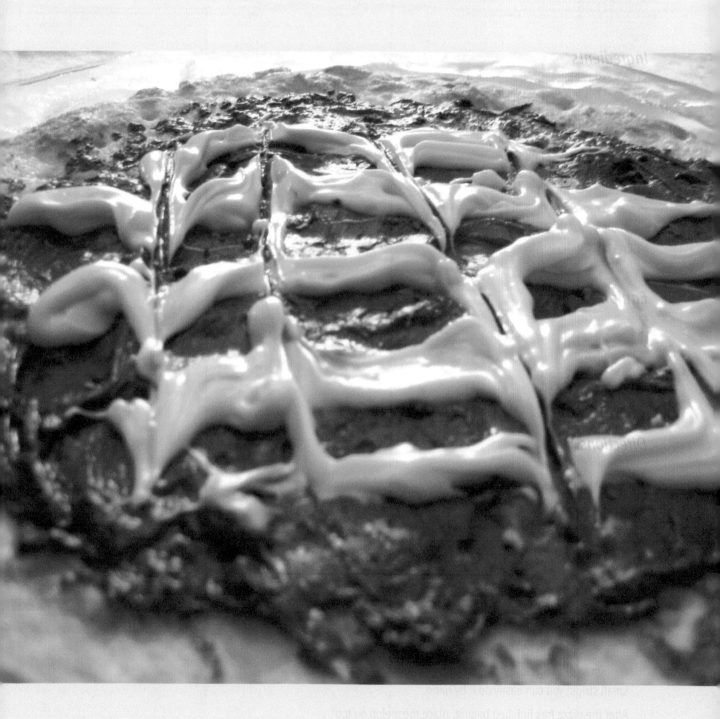

Servings: 4 – 6
Prep time: 5 minutes
Cooking time: 10 minutes
Cost: 4.08

Ingredients
1 plain pre-made 12" thin crust pizza
1 cup of Nutella
1/4 cup melted white chocolate morsels

Equipment
Baking sheet
Measuring cups
Parchment paper (optional)
Spoon for making a design on the pizza

Directions
1. Pre-heat the oven according to the directions
    on the pizza crust package.
    Spread the Nutella evenly over the crust and
    bake for 8 minutes.

2. While the pizza is baking, melt ¼ cup of
    white chocolate in a microwave-safe bowl
    for about 50-60 seconds (until the chips
    have begun to melt).

3. Remove the pizza from the oven and drizzle
    the white chocolate sauce over the pizza.
    Using the back of a spoon, make a design on
    the top of the pizza as pictured above.
    This is a great place to get creative and
    decorate the dish in a style of your choosing.

SMOKED SALMON PIZZA

Ellen had her first smoked salmon pizza in 1992 at Wolfgang Puck's first restaurant, Spago, in Los Angeles. It was cutting edge at the time—not surprising for Wolfgang Puck. We've reinvented it here for you to enjoy at home. Cut this into small bite size pieces for a wonderful appetizer.

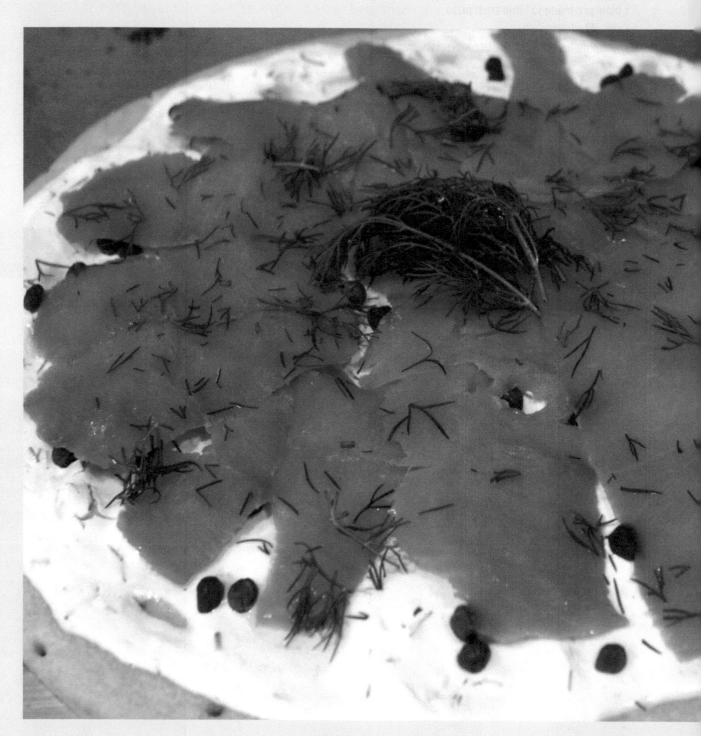

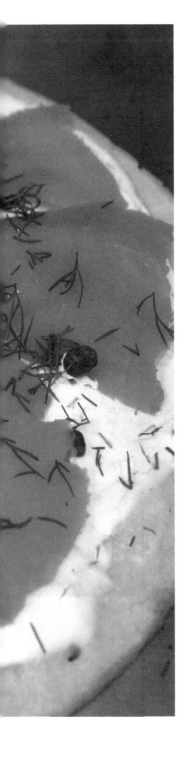

Ingredients

8 oz. smoked salmon
¼ cup large capers
1 tablespoon lemon juice + extra for sprinkling on final pizza
½ teaspoon wasabi paste
    (Japanese horseradish, comes in tubes)
1 cup sour cream
1 tablespoon chopped dill + extra for sprinkling on final pizza
1 premade pizza crust
Olive oil for brushing the crust (about 2 tablespoons)

Equipment

Baking sheet
Mixing bowl
Measuring cups & spoons

Directions

1. Follow the package directions for preheating oven
   to bake the pizza.
   Brush pizza lightly with olive oil.

2. In a small mixing bowl mix the sour cream,
   lemon juice, dill, and wasabi.
   Spread this evenly over the crust.
   Top with capers and bake for 8 – 10 minutes.

3. Once the pizza has finished baking, place
   the smoked salmon on the pizza, covering
   it entirely.
   Sprinkle the entire pizza with fresh dill and
   lemon juice.

This base is baked. Salmon is added after baking.

Servings: 4 – 6
Prep time: 5 minutes
Cooking time: 10 minutes
Cost: $15.16

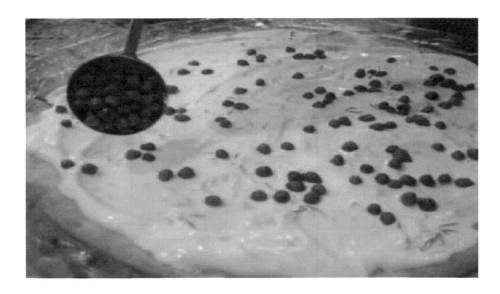

PESTO PIZZA

This mouth-wateringly delicious pizza hits all the right taste buds with the pesto-parmesan-tomato combination. Great for a summer picnic lunch or a late night exam break, this pizza is sure to disappear almost as soon as it's served!

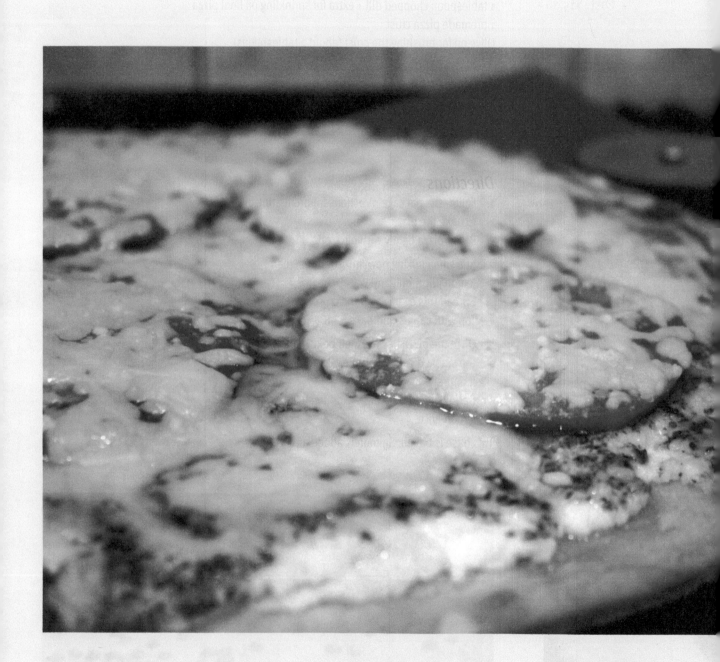

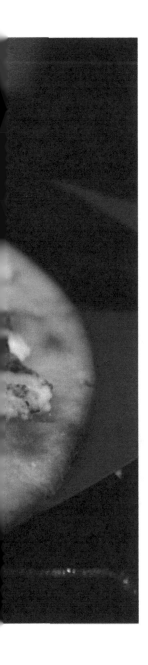

Servings: 4 – 6
Prep time: 10 minutes
Cooking time: 10 minutes
Cost: $14.45

Ingredients
1 large ripe tomato, sliced thickly
1 cup shredded mozzarella
1 cup ricotta cheese
½ cup parmesan cheese

Pesto Sauce Ingredients
1 cup basil leaves
2 tablespoons pine nuts
¼ cup olive oil
½ cup grated parmesan
¼ teaspoon of pepper
1 teaspoon garlic paste

Equipment
Baking sheet (optional)
Mixing bowl
Paring knife

Directions
1. Prepare the pizza crust according to package directions.

2. Slice the tomato.

3. Make sure the ricotta is soft enough to be spread, and spread it over the base of the crust.

4. In a blender, combine the pesto sauce ingredients and then spread the finished pesto sauce over the ricotta.

5. Place the tomato over the pesto. Sprinkle with the Parmesan and mozzarella.

6. Bake for 8 – 10 minutes, according to package directions.

Tuna Artichoke Pizza

For a taste of authentic Italian flavors, try this unique tribute to an original pizza recipe Sophia encountered in Rome. The tomatoes will burst in your mouth as the tender artichoke and tuna unite to form a creamy, sharp taste you won't forget.

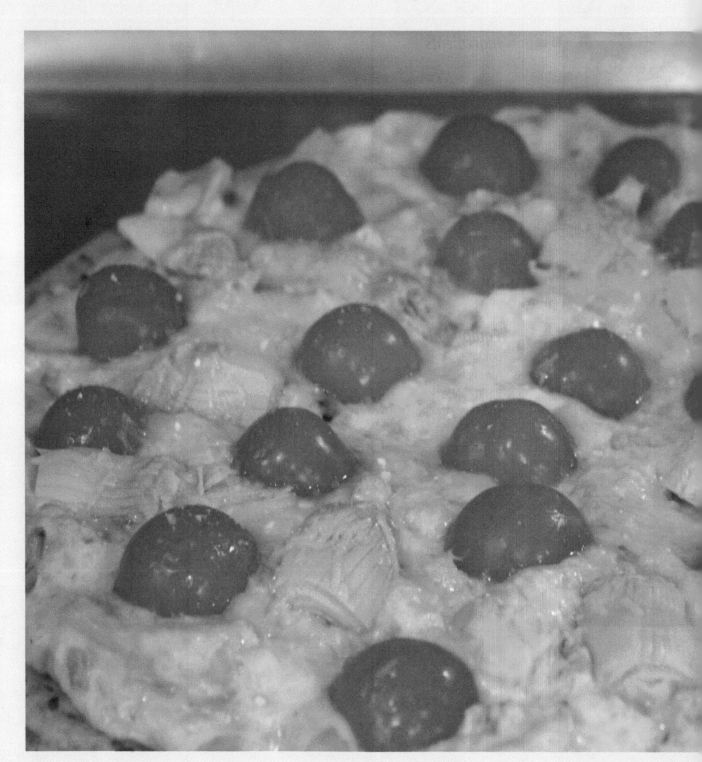

Servings: 4 – 6
Prep time: 10 minutes
Cooking time: 15 minutes
Cost: $7.72

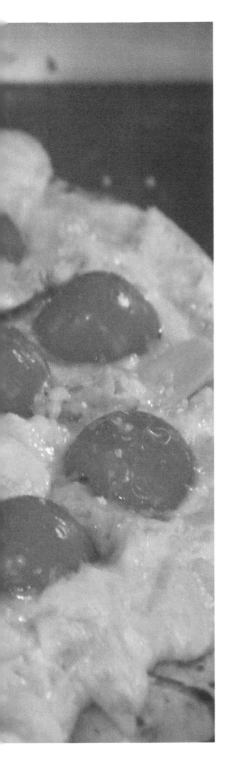

Ingredient
1 prepared pizza crust
10 cherry tomatoes, cut in half
1 x 14 oz. can artichoke hearts, quartered
2 tablespoons Parmesan cheese
Béchamel sauce (see below)

Béchamel Sauce Ingredients
1 cup milk
2 tablespoons olive oil
2 tablespoons flour
1/2 cup parmesan cheese
1 tablespoon lemon juice
¼ teaspoon ground nutmeg
½ teaspoon salt
½ teaspoon ground black pepper
1 x 5 oz. can tuna fish, drained

Equipment
Medium size saucepan for béchamel sauce
Baking sheet
Measuring cups & spoons

Directions
1. Follow the package directions for preheating oven to bake the pizza. Brush pizza lightly with olive oil.

2. Whisk olive oil and flour in a saucepan over medium heat until the mixture has become incorporated and has a blond color, about 2 minutes.

3. Slowly whisk in the milk. Heat over medium-high, bringing the sauce to a light boil.

4. Once it boils, turn the heat down to medium-low and cook until thickened, whisking occasionally for 5 – 6 minutes.

5. Turn the heat off and add tuna, ½ cup of Parmesan, lemon juice, salt, pepper, and nutmeg to the sauce. Spread over the pizza crust.

6. Top with artichoke hearts and grape tomatoes, distributing evenly, then sprinkle with 2 tablespoons Parmesan.

7. Bake in oven for approximately 8 – 10 minutes.

MAKE YOUR OWN PIZZA PARTY

This is a very fun party. Have a variety of toppings for your friends to choose from—alternatively you could ask each person to bring 1 item for topping pizzas.

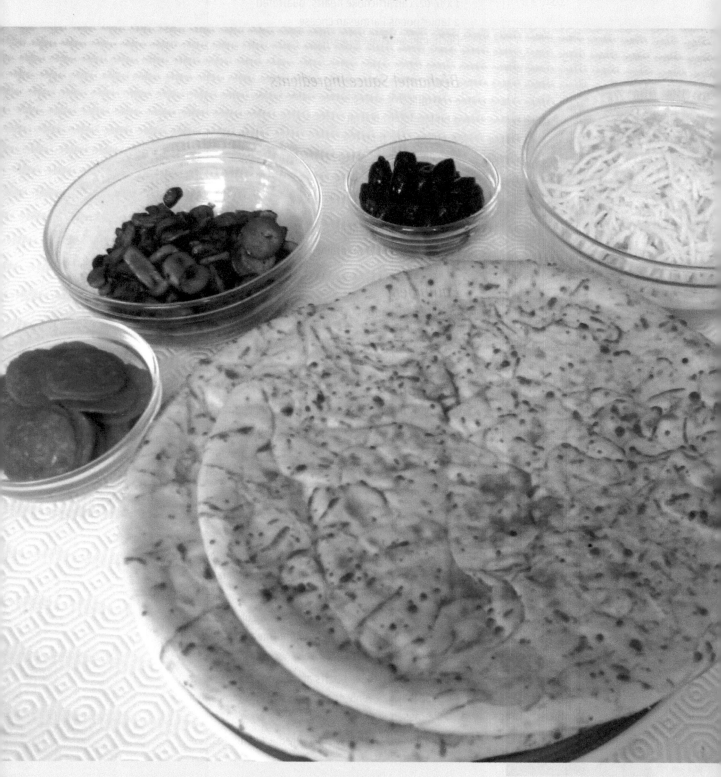

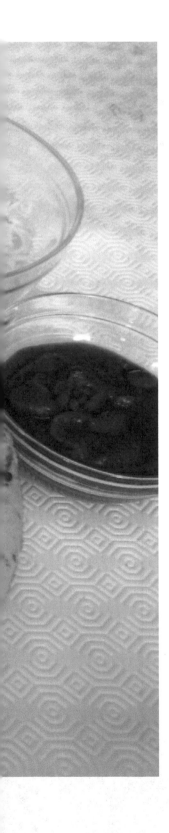

Sample Ingredient List
Premade pizza crusts
Pizza sauce
Mushrooms
Onions
Pepperoni
Peppers
Olives
Feta/goat cheese
Shredded mozzarella cheese
Parmesan cheese
Pesto
Etc. Etc. Etc.

Equipment
Baking sheets or pizza stones
Bowls for presenting ingredients

Directions
Preheat oven and prepare crust
according to package directions.
Top with your favorite sauce and
toppings and bake.

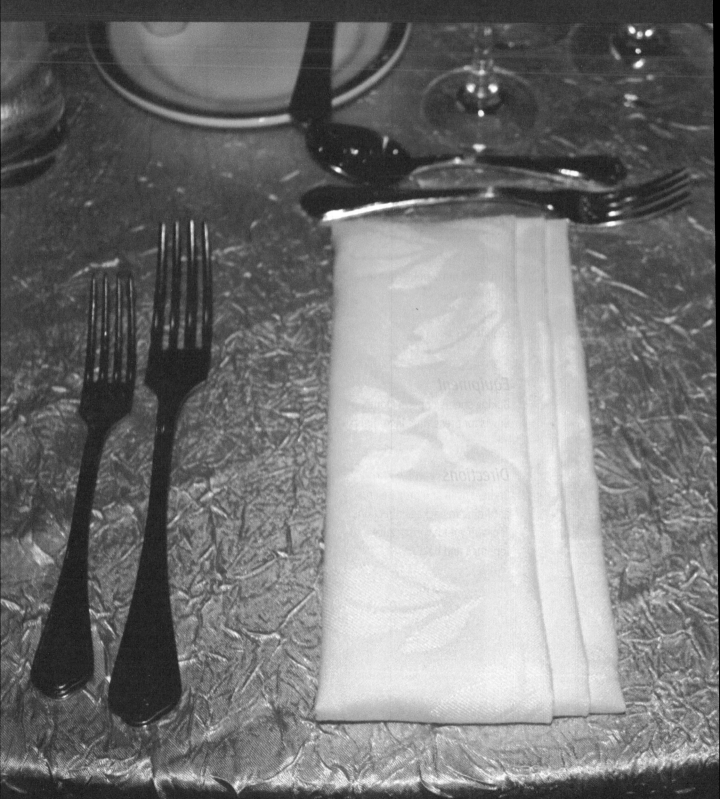

14. Epicurean Etiquette

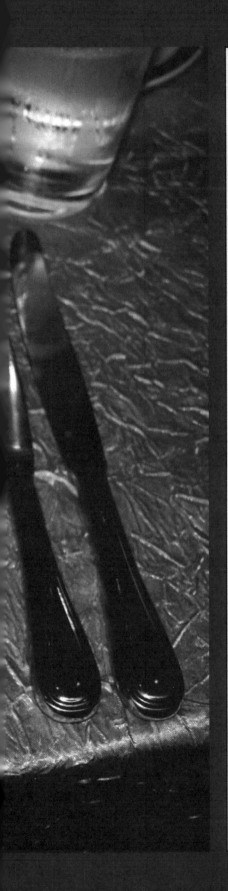

Epicurean Etiquette

Which fork is for salad? Is soup for slurping or sipping? If you have ever wanted to host an elegant dinner party for your friends but find yourself settling for disposable meals; if you have ever thought of hosting a tea party on a rainy afternoon: have no fear! From serving proper tea to setting a table, this section will teach you how to wow your guests with a classy affair to be remembered.

Setting and Serving

Don't be flustered by formality! In reality, it's just a code that you can learn. With our easy tricks, you will never get the table-setting jitters again. We'll walk you through tabletop basics all the way through to the dreaded arrangement of silverware. We have included a picture of a basic place setting to help you with visualizing our guidelines. If you'd like to bring the level of formality down a notch, simply leave out such items as the butter plate and knife. Just keep in mind that you will still want to be practicing good serving habits no matter who is seated at your table!

Tabletop Tips

So before you start worrying about misplaced silverware, let's talk about the table itself. Whether it's a formal dinner with a professor or a laid back evening with friends, it's always good to have either a tablecloth or place mats (or both, if you're feeling inspired!). This decreases the chance of spilled food or liquid permanently staining your tabletop. It also adds a nice splash of color or design to the meal. Make sure that everything is measured out evenly—that is, keep the centerpiece in the actual center and make sure people's seats are evenly spaced. Why a centerpiece? It's a fun way to add a holiday or special occasion theme to the meal, and it draws everyone's attention to the center, the conversation at hand, and (of course) the food!

Dish Drama

Having anxiety attacks over where to put which dish? Relax; it's a lot simpler than it may seem. The service plate faces the diner. The butter plate should be to the left of a person's place setting, above the forks. Save the dessert plate until it's time for dessert. Some people like to put the appetizer dish on top of the main course dish, but we suggest avoiding this practice if possible. That way, you will avoid some likely spills. In general, you want to bring the plate for the course to be served just before serving it or with the food already on it. Serve from the left side of your guests (being careful not to disturb them), and remove from the right side. Wineglasses should be arranged by size—descending or ascending, take your pick!

Silverware Standards

Arranging the silverware in proper order may seem like a daunting task, and rightfully so. Never fear, though; the most essential secret is about to be yours. Ready? The correct way to use silverware at your setting is to start from the outside and work your way inward. In the same way, you should set the table with the silverware that will be used last closest to the plate and the silverware to be used first furthest out. Forks should always be on the left, with the meat fork to the left of the salad fork and the salad fork to the left of the entrée fork. If fish is to be served, the fish fork should be to the left of the meat fork. The knife should be closest to the plate on the right side, with soup or and/or fruit spoons outside and the oyster fork just outside of the fruit spoon. The butter knife should be set at a diagonal at the top of the butter plate, as you might expect. As a general rule, you never want to place more than three of any utensil (with the exception of forks, which may increase in number depending on what you're serving). Best not to overdo it and intimidate your guests! If you're feeling ambitious and plan to serve more than three courses prior to dessert, bring the fourth fork in with its corresponding course. Finally, bring whatever utensil the dessert requires on the dessert plate before it's served.

Mealtime Manners

We have a secret to share: you do not need to be a stiff-backed, delicate, cautious diner with a protruding pinky finger In order to behave with grace and decorum at a meal! Whether you're dining for 5 or 500 dollars a plate, these simple tips will imbue you with the elegance you need to ingest with finesse.

Before you breeze by these rules or save them until 1 hour prior to the big dinner with the future in-laws, keep in mind that the best way to be prepared for any dining situation is to practice good habits wherever you are. So try not to slouch or shovel your food in at the cafeteria (unless you are really in a hurry); not only do poor posture and overzealous eating strain the digestive process, but they build a sloppy default dining setting into your body. If you find yourself in a stressful or tense situation, you may revert to these no-no's without even realizing what you are actually doing! Remember that the way you behave at the table reflects on yourself and also signals respect (or a lack thereof!) to your partner.
Instead of explaining each and every rule of etiquette in painstaking detail (both impractical and, let's admit it, a bit boring!), we have decided to clue you in to the most important rules. These basic guidelines will serve you well at any situation in which you find yourself and will be easy enough to remember that you can work them into your daily routine in a very short time! Please, try not to be mortified if you realize as you read this list that you have been guilty of violating some major etiquette standards. We will stand by the 'ignorance is innocence' policy and let you off the hook this time.

What To Do With Your Body

1. Do not chew with your mouth open

All right, so we know your parents have been badgering you with this line since before you even had teeth—with good reason! If you have ever eaten with someone who displays everything happening inside his or her mouth, you must know how unpleasant it can be. Try to spare others this unappetizing habit.

2. Do not speak with food in your mouth

Like the first rule, this one may seem obvious and already ingrained into your etiquette memory bank. Yet the number of people who inadvertently make conversation while working on a meal may surprise you. Needless to say, pre-chewed food decorating the tablecloth makes for a less than aesthetically appealing dinnertime sight. In order to avoid the trap of being caught off-guard, see the following rule.

3. Eat slowly and take small bites

"What? Small bites? But the food is so good, I must get as much of it into my mouth as possible!" There are numerous excuses like that one (some people take large bites when they're nervous, others because they're famished, etc.), but none of those excuses is legitimate when it comes to dining decorum. Firstly, it's actually not good for you to stuff huge portions of food in your mouth all at once. You're less likely to chew properly and more likely to give your digestive tract a difficult task. And we won't even get into heartburn or the myriad other negative side effects of chomping off a fistful of food or eating at breakneck pace. If you intend to be a good dinnertime companion, you won't be able to keep up a steady conversation if you always have huge portions in your mouth that take several minutes to chew through properly. You will also find that you can savor the taste better and eat less while still eating enough—if you take your time. So remember, slow down and eat little portions.

4. Elbows off when you can

We know that this rule can be annoying and out of some outdated era when women still wore corsets and men held the doors open for ladies. Still, the origin of this time-old custom has some element of logic. If you are leaning on your elbows, you are likely hunching over and not sitting straight. Like we explained earlier, we are not telling you to be stiff and straight. But you must know by now that hunching over is terrible for your back, and (you guessed it!) not that great for digesting, either. It may seem at first that you will feel more relaxed if you lean over and put the weight on your elbows, but your forearms are just as good. Try leaning against the back of the chair or resting on your forearms when need be. You will begin to feel a difference in no time.

5. Do not invade other people's dining space

This may appear to be an odd suggestion, but a shameful number of people mistakenly make their dining partners uncomfortable by being inconsiderate. All it takes is an elbow sticking out while vigorously cutting a piece of meat, and your next-door neighbor is being tenderized as you slice. Try, if you can, to keep your elbows down when cutting or when bringing food to your mouth. Try not to sit in such a way that you deprive someone next to you or across from you of any legroom. Avoid reaching over the table without asking for someone to pass you what you are reaching for. If you have already begun to reach, be sure to pardon yourself and refrain from doing so again!

What To Do With Your Cutlery

1. Don't wave around your cutlery

   Even if you are giving a passionate speech about the lessons learned by mankind over the history of civilization, do not use your cutlery to make your point clearer. Some of us tend to gesticulate when talking—do not make it a habit to use your silverware as an extension of yourself! Try not to point at people with your knife, either; not only is it rude, but it may just be a bit frightening.

2. Once it's off the table, keep it off

   The rule with silverware is that once you have removed it from the table for use, you never put it back on the table. That way, you avoid offending your guests, hosts, or restaurant owners by staining the tablecloth with whatever food is on your cutlery. Always return it to the plate. See the following rule for more information on how to signal what stage of the meal you're on.

3. Silverware sign language

   So you need to take a restroom break or answer an urgent phone call. Politely excuse yourself without drawing too much attention to what you are doing. Before you get up, place your silverware in the 'I'm returning/I'm not done yet' position: cross the fork, prongs down, over the knife to form a wide angle opening towards you. To indicate that you're done with the course: place the knife, blade facing you, and the fork, prongs down again, in a diagonal across your plate and at about 4 o'clock and 10 o'clock. The knife and fork should be parallel to one another.

4. Don't bite

   Well you can bite your food, but please refrain at all costs from biting your silverware, glass, or cup. Enough said.

5. Don't make unpleasant noises

   Aside from biting, there is a whole host of other noises you can accidentally make over the course of your meal. Scraping the plate while cutting your food, clanging silverware together or on the plate, scraping at a bowl with your spoon, slurping or gulping loudly, belching, and the list goes on. Whatever you do, try to eat and drink with grace and to be attentive to the sounds you're making.

TEA PARTY FOR 10

Have 10 of your closest friends over for tea. It's easy and quick with these tea sandwich recipes and shortcuts. We recommend making 7 of each type of sandwich, for a total of 21 sandwiches. This gives each person 2 sandwiches. Serve sandwiches with store-bought cookies and hot tea. If it's a warm summer day, you may want to offer your guests iced tea as well. Our recipe for sweet southern tea follows.

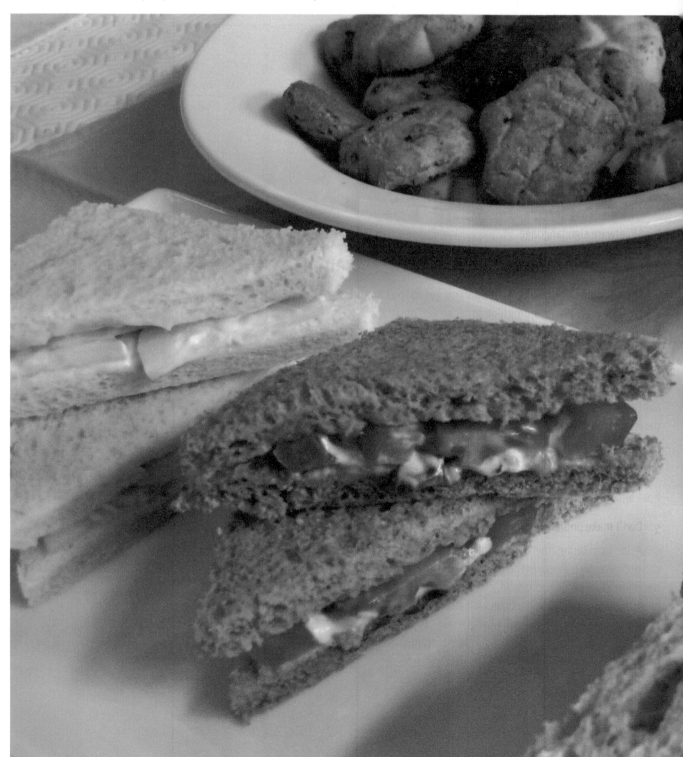

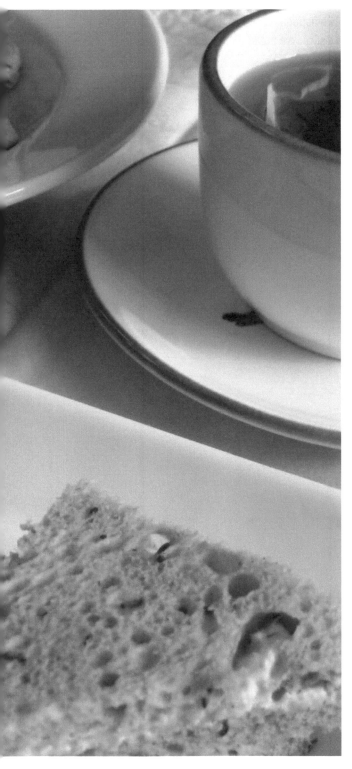

Teatime Tips

Serving tea has been a human custom for thousands of years. In the Epicurean Etiquette section, we give you tips on hosting a memorable tea party for your friends. We want to give you a brief idea of what range of teas you ought to have available and what type of food goes with them. Tea has been known to provide salutary health effects and comes in a wide variety of flavors to cater to all tastes.

Herbal Tea

This type of tea includes what are commonly referred to as fruit teas. The 'herbal' or 'fruit' element of the name derives from the process of infusing the tea with herbs or fruit to give it a distinct flavor. As you might imagine, these teas often have a light and fruity taste to them. They help to balance more savory flavors, so you might want to serve them with sandwiches.

Black Teas

These full-bodied teas tend to be smokier and stronger in flavor. Sometimes, people dull the heaviness with milk and sugar or honey. Popular black teas such as Earl Grey and Prince of Wales are often served in the morning with breakfast. They also go well with biscuits and cookies and are ideal for dunking.

Green Teas

Known for their bitterness, the green teas originated in China and made their way around the world. Many people have begun to flock to green tea usage, hoping to reap some of the health benefits widely associated with green tea. Although the bitter taste can be intimidating at first, you may find that if you endure, you will discover intricate layers of flavor.

Cucumber on White with Lemon Mayonnaise

Ingredients

1 large cucumber, peeled and sliced in
　　about ¼ inch slices
½ cup mayonnaise
1 tablespoon lemon juice
1/2 teaspoon salt
¼ teaspoon black pepper
14 slices white bread

Equipment

Cutting board
Mixing bowl
Measuring cups & spoons

Directions

1. Peel and slice the cucumbers.

2. Mix the mayo with the lemon juice, salt, and pepper.

3. Trim the crust off the bread (you can save it for bread pudding or panzanella salad if you wish). Line up your slices of bread and spread a small amount of mayo on each slice, top one slice of bread with 4-5 slices of cucumber, top with another piece of bread and cut in half on the diagonal.

We've recommended different bread for each sandwich but feel free to choose your favorite breads—you can use all white if you choose or pumpernickel instead of rye for the smoked salmon.

Prep time: 5 minutes
Cooking time: 0 minutes
Servings: 10
Cost: $3.61

Smoked Salmon on Rye

Ingredients

4 oz. cream cheese
2 oz. smoked salmon (half a package)
2 tablespoons lemon juice
1 tablespoon fresh dill
¼ teaspoon black pepper
14 slices rye bread

Equipment

2 cup food processor
Measuring spoons

Directions

1. Place all ingredients, except the bread, in a food processor and blend until well combined.

2. Remove crusts from the bread. Spread a good amount of the salmon cream cheese on a slice of bread, cover with another slice of bread and cut on a diagonal.

Prep time: 10 minutes
Cooking time: 0 minutes
Servings: 10
Cost: $8.49

Tomato on Wheat with Basil Mayonnaise

Ingredients
2 large tomatoes
½ cup mayonnaise
½ cup basil leaves
½ teaspoon salt
¼ teaspoon black pepper
14 slices of wheat bread

Equipment
Mixing bowl
Measuring cups & spoons
Cutting board & knife (preferably serrated for cutting tomatoes)

Directions
1. Slice the tomatoes into ½ inch slices.

2. Cut the crust off the bread.

3. Shred the basil leaves by hand and add to the mayo. Add the salt and pepper and mix well. Spread a small amount on each slice of bread.

4. Place 1 tomato slice on a piece of bread, top with another piece of bread and slice diagonally.

Prep time: 5 minutes
Cooking time: 0 minutes
Servings: 10
Cost: $5.26

Sweet Southern Iced Tea

You can ice any type of tea, but we recommend using an herbal tea for this recipe. Herbal teas, especially fruit teas, take well to the sweetening process and already often have a natural sweetness of their own.

Ingredients
4 – 5 bags herbal tea
1 quart water
4 tablespoons sugar
Ice cubes (about 6)

Equipment
Boiling pot or electric kettle
Strainer (if using bags without strings)

Directions
Bring the water to a boil. Turn the heat off and add the sugar, then add the tea bags and allow them to steep for about 8 – 10 minutes. Be sure not to let the strings fall into the pot! Remove the tea bags once they have finished infusing the hot water and squeeze to make sure you have gotten all the juice out that you can—A secret we have is to spoon the bag, then wrap the string around the spoon and pull.

Transfer the pot of tea to a large plastic container, add the ice cubes, and refrigerate for at least 2 hours.

You can also serve this hot, but we prefer iced for the summertime.

15. ENTERTAINING BY CITY:
LESS THAN $10 A HEAD

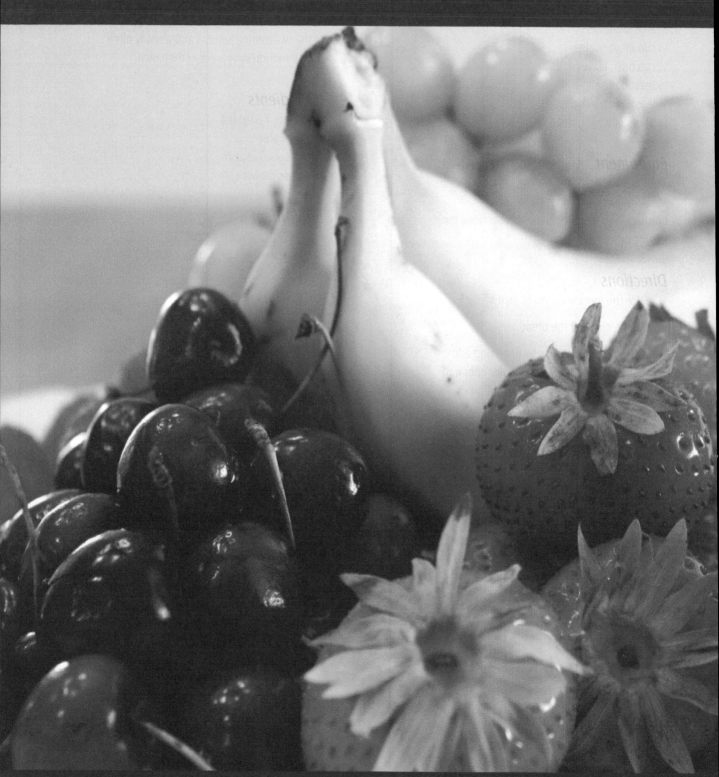

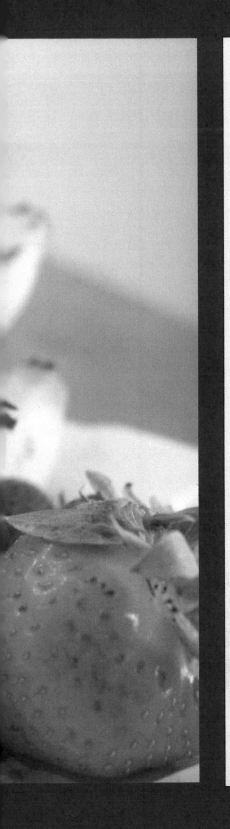

Dinner parties for 4

Naples, Italy $6.33 per person

Istanbul, Turkey $8.31 per person

New Orleans, Louisiana $9.16 per person

Athens, Greece $9.47 per person

Santa Fe, New Mexico $9.84 per person

THE NAPLES DINNER
$6.33 PER PERSON

The menu:
Artichoke Bruschetta
Penne Puttanesca
Mascarpone Berry Cocktail

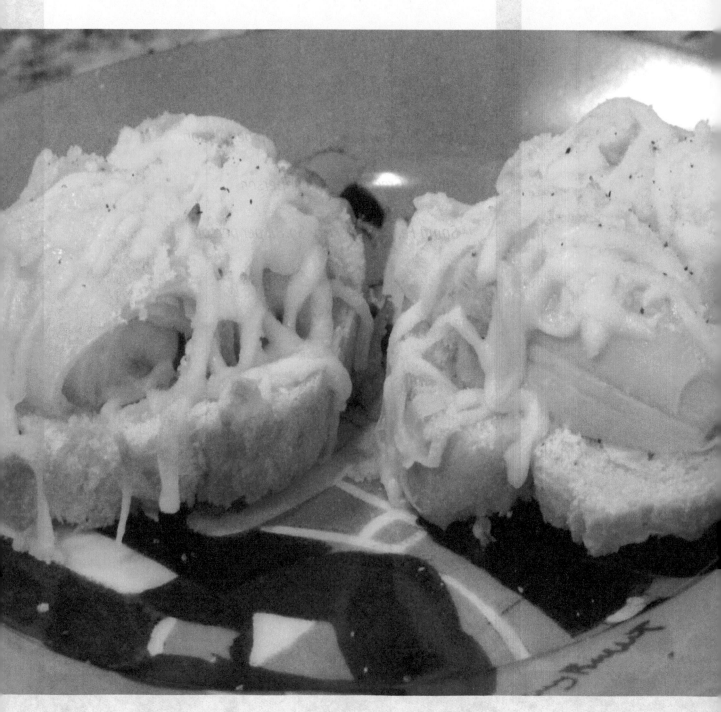

ARTICHOKE BRUSCHETTA

Bruschetta has its origins in Italy and dates back to the 15th century. The original recipe was grilled bread rubbed with garlic and drizzled with salt, pepper, and olive oil.
Today bruschetta has the same base of grilled or toasted bread but add any topping you like. Use your leftover artichoke hearts to make Artichoke Pesto Alfredo Pasta.

Servings: 4
Prep time: 5 minutes
Cooking time: 8 minutes
Cost: $7.23

Ingredients

1/3 loaf French bread (2 slices per person)
1 can artichoke hearts, contains 6-7 whole hearts
1 tablespoon shredded mozzarella per slice
½ teaspoon grated Parmesan per slice
1 clove garlic, cut in half
Olive oil
Freshly ground black pepper

Equipment

Baking sheet
Serrated knife for slicing bread
Measuring cups & spoons
Parchment paper (optional, for easy cleanup)

Directions

1. Preheat oven to 400 degrees F.

2. Cut the bread into ½ inch thick slices. Place on a baking sheet covered with parchment paper and drizzle with olive oil. Bake for 3 minutes in the oven.

3. If the artichoke hearts are already quartered, leave them as they are, otherwise cut each heart in 4 pieces.

4. After the bread has come out of the oven, cut the end of a clove of garlic off and brush the bread with the exposed end (see Basic Bruschetta recipe in Finger Foods for a photo of this technique). Layer the bread slices with approximately 2-3 slices of artichoke and sprinkle with shredded mozzarella, grated Parmesan, and black pepper. Bake for 5 minutes at 400 degrees F. Drizzle with olive oil and serve immediately.

PENNE PUTTANESCA

Another classic Italian dish very popular in the U.S. It's a spicy pasta dish with a tomato sauce.

Servings: 4
Prep time: 10 minutes
Cooking time: 15 minutes
Cost: $7.12

Ingredients

1 pound penne pasta
28 oz. can diced tomatoes
6 oz. can large olives, drained
1 yellow onion, diced
1 jar capers (3.5 ounce), drained
¼ teaspoon cayenne pepper
1 tablespoon garlic paste
1 tablespoon tomato paste
2 tablespoons olive oil
2 teaspoons salt

Equipment

Pasta pot
Large sauté pan for making the sauce
Colander
Cutting board
Measuring spoons

Directions

1. Cook pasta according to package directions. When the water has boiled, salt generously (using 2 - 3 tablespoons of salt).

2. While the pasta is cooking dice the onion.

3. Meanwhile heat a sauté pan over medium heat. Once the pan is hot add 2 tablespoons of olive oil. Add the cayenne and onion to the pan and cook for 2 – 3 minutes on medium. Then proceed to add the can of tomatoes, but do not drain! The juice from the can will help to create a good consistency for the sauce. Bring the sauce to a boil over medium heat.

4. While the sauce is boiling, drain the olives and the capers. Add the capers, olives, tomato paste, garlic paste, and salt to the sauce. Cook for 10 minutes over medium-low to allow the flavors to marry.

5. Add the pasta to the sauté pan and mix thoroughly. Sprinkle each dish with grated Parmesan and serve.

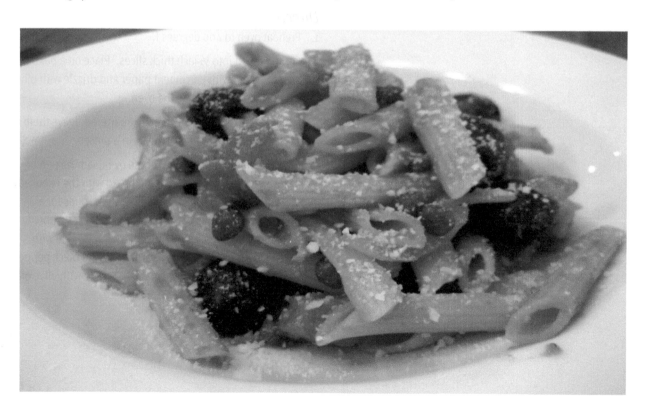

MASCARPONE BERRY COCKTAIL

We have a light dessert for you to finish your Italian dinner. Mascarpone is Italian cream cheese. It's a little richer than cream cheese you'll find here and is a wonderful accessory for fresh berries.

Servings: 4
Prep time: 1 minute
Cooking time: 0
Cost: $11.64

Ingredients
½ pint fresh raspberries
½ pint fresh blackberries
8 oz. mascarpone
    (comes in 8 oz tubs)
1 teaspoon lime juice
1 teaspoon vanilla extract
Lime zest for sprinkling
    (optional)

Equipment
Mixing bowl
Cocktail glasses

Directions
1. Let the mascarpone soften on the counter for about an hour.

2. Once soft, add the mascarpone to a mixing bowl.

3. Using a fork mix thoroughly with lime juice and vanilla extract.

4. Place the berries into a cocktail glass, top with the mascarpone and serve!

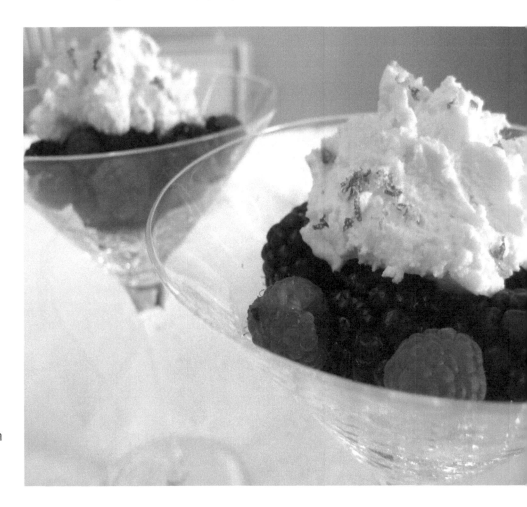

ISTANBUL DINNER
$8.31 PER PERSON

The menu:
Imam Bayildi with Cicak and Pita
Lamb with Yogurt and Tomato
Turkish Delight

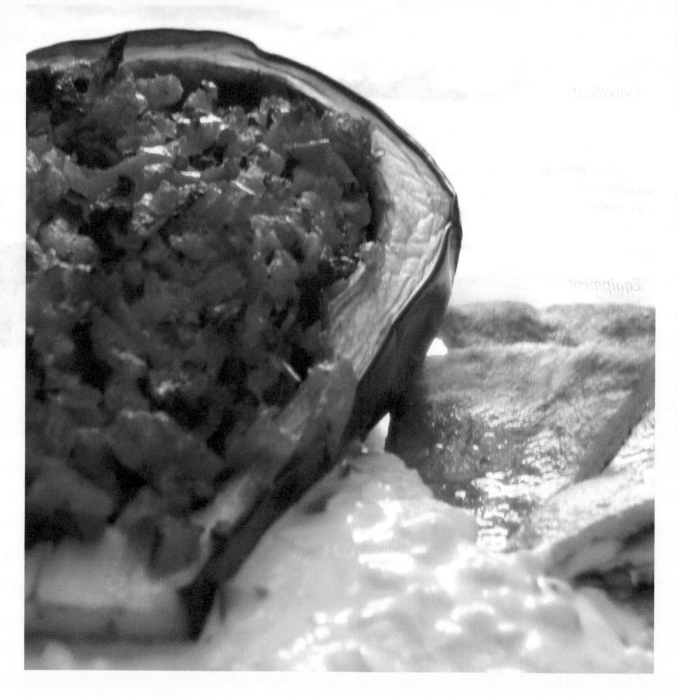

IMAM BAYILDI WITH CICAK AND PITA

Oh yes, this is as decadent as it looks. Turkish food is so flavorful you'll experience a flavor explosion in every bite. This is a meal you'll soon have cravings for.

Ingredients
2 eggplants (about 6 inches long each)
2 tablespoons olive oil
1 large onion, chopped
1 tablespoon garlic paste
¼ cup lemon juice
5 peeled chopped tomatoes
       (peeled and whole, available in cans)
1 small red pepper, diced and seeded
1 zucchini, diced
3 tablespoons fresh parsley, chopped
1 teaspoon salt
½ teaspoon black pepper

Cicak Ingredients
2 cups plain Greek yogurt
2 tablespoons garlic paste
3 teaspoons lemon juice
1 large cucumber, diced
1 teaspoon salt

Equipment
Sauté pan
Baking sheet

Prep time: 20 minutes
Cooking time: 1 hr. 10 minutes
Servings: 4
Cost: $15.52

Directions
Preheat the oven to 350 degrees F.

To make the imam bayildi:
Cut each eggplant in half lengthwise and scoop out the center of each half and reserve the eggplant from the center. Drizzle the eggplant halves with olive oil, place on a baking sheet, and fill generously with the filling. Bake at 350 for 1 hour.

To make the filling for the imam bayildi:
In a sauté pan over medium heat, allow the onions, pepper, and zucchini to soften in 2 table-spoons of olive oil, about 5 minutes. Add the garlic paste and stir for about 1 minute, then add the tomatoes, leftover eggplant meat (chopped), and parsley. Season the mix with 1 teaspoon of salt and ½ teaspoon of black pepper, stir, and sauté for another 2 – 3 minutes. Remove from the heat.

To make the cicak:
Mix the ingredients for cicak together in a bowl and serve with the Imam bayildi and freshly toasted pita bread for a delicious first course.

LAMB WITH YOGURT AND TOMATO

*A Mediterranean Middle Eastern delight in every bite.
Don't be intimidated by all the steps in this recipe---you can
do them simultaneously and the end result is so delicious
it's worth having to clean 3 pans! Your friends will be wowed
by how authentic and flavorful this dish is.*

Servings: 4
Prep time: 1 hour 10 minutes
Cooking time: 20 minutes
Cost: $13.42

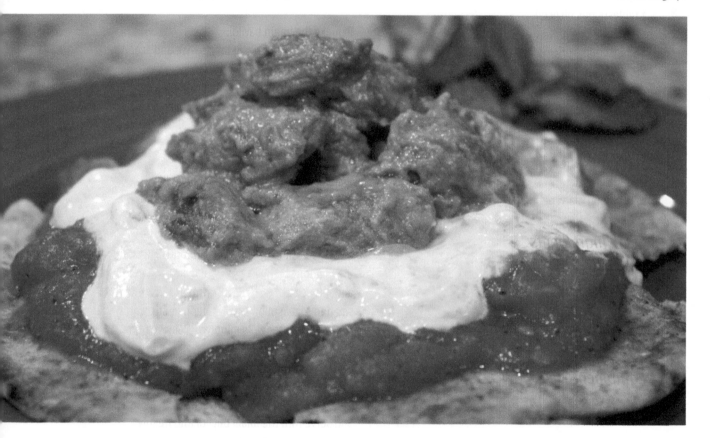

Ingredients
1 lb. lean lamb meat (stew meat)
4 pieces of pita bread (+ 1 tablespoon olive oil
for brushing pita)
Tomatoes (see below)
Yogurt (see below)
Lamb Marinade (see below)

Tomato Ingredients
28 ounce can of diced tomatoes
1 teaspoon garlic paste
½ teaspoon ground black pepper

Yogurt Ingredients
1 cup Greek yogurt
½ teaspoon salt
½ teaspoon paprika
¼ cup sautéed pine nuts (pignoli nuts)

Marinade Ingredients
½ cup plain Greek yogurt
1 onion, chopped or grated
1 teaspoon salt
1/8 teaspoon cayenne pepper
¼ teaspoon garlic powder

Equipment
Mixing bowls
2 large sauté pans for cooking lamb and tomatoes
Small sauté pan for toasting the pine nuts
Chopping board & knife
Measuring cups & spoons

Directions
1 Hour before cooking, prepare the marinade:
In a medium-sized mixing bowl, combine the ½ cup of yogurt, grated onion, salt, cayenne, and garlic powder. Mix thoroughly, then add the lamb and stir until the meat is fully coated. Cover the bowl with plastic wrap and marinate in the fridge for 1 hour.

When you are ready to cook:
Preheat oven to 350 degrees F for the pita bread.

Heat a large sauté pan with 2 tablespoons of olive oil and sauté the meat and what's left of the marinade on medium-high heat for 12 minutes, ensuring that the lamb retains its juiciness and has a tender consistency.

While the meat is cooking, cook the tomatoes and pita. Brush each pita with 1 teaspoon of olive oil, sprinkle with a pinch of salt, and place in the oven for 2 minutes or toast in a conventional toaster oven until the bread begins to brown. Remove and break the pita into large chunks directly onto the dishes you intend to serve on.

For the tomatoes: Add the tomatoes to a sauté pan and cook for about 15 minutes on medium heat with a teaspoon of garlic paste and ½ teaspoon of ground black pepper.

For the yogurt: toast the pine nuts on medium-low heat in a small dry sauté pan for 1 – 2 minutes (until they are tan in color)---remember to never walk away from nuts toasting in a pan—they can burn very quickly. In a separate bowl, mix the yogurt with ½ teaspoon of salt, ½ teaspoon of paprika, and the pine nuts.

This dish is plated in layers as follows:
PITA
TOMATOES
YOGURT
LAMB

Garnish the plate with mint leaves and serve piping hot!

TURKISH DELIGHT

Find authentic Turkish Delight at your local Mediterranean store or restaurant. Alternatively, you can purchase it in advance online from several reliable sites. Arrange on a platter and serve with a light herbal tea for a satisfyingly sweet end to your meal.

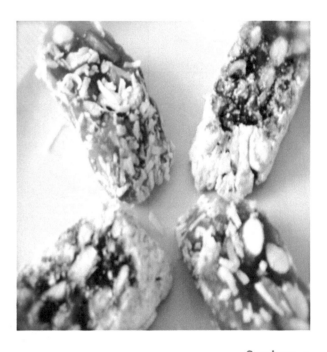

Servings: 4
Prep time: 5 minutes
Cooking time: 0 minutes
Cost: $4.29

The New Orleans Dinner
$9.16 per person

The menu:
Oysters Rockefeller Tarts
Chicken and Sausage Gumbo
Bananas Foster Ice Cream

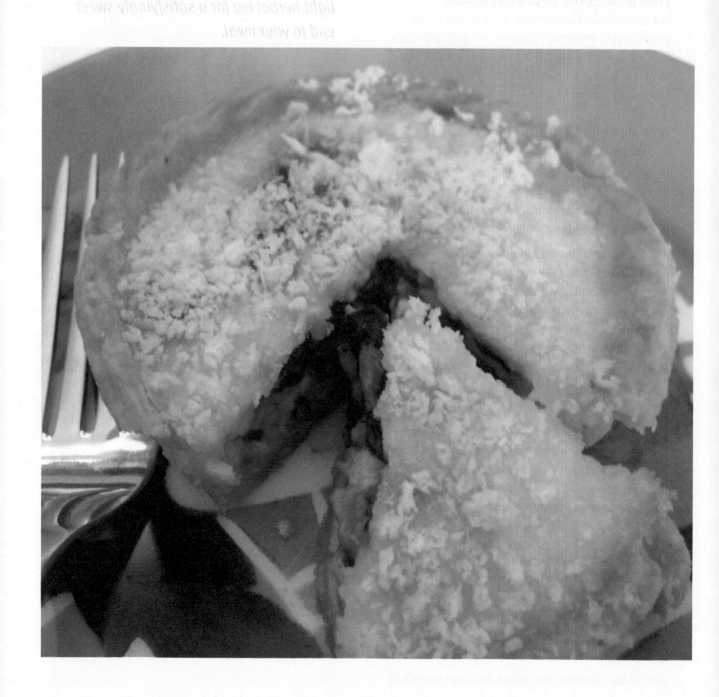

OYSTERS ROCKEFELLER TARTS

This is our take on oysters Rockefeller. It's a great first course for this New Orleans dinner. Layers of sautéed oysters, spinach and custard with a crunchy top make for an incredible flavor and texture sensation.

Servings: 4
Prep time: 10 minutes
Cooking time: 35 minutes
Cost: $12.89

Ingredients

8 oz. container of fresh oysters
6 oz. bag of washed spinach
1 package of pastry shells
    (comes in packs of 8 in the frozen section near
    puff pastry)
½ cup heavy cream
2 eggs
¼ cup Parmesan
¼ cup bread crumbs (preferably Panko)
4 tablespoons of olive oil, divided
2 teaspoons garlic paste
1 teaspoon salt
½ teaspoon black pepper

Equipment

Large sauté pan
Baking sheet
Mixing bowls
Measuring cups and spoons
Parchment paper (optional)

Directions

1. Preheat the oven to 375 degrees F.

2. Thaw the pastry shells according to package directions. Place on a baking sheet.

3. Mix the Parmesan cheese and bread crumbs in a small bowl. In a separate bowl mix the cream and eggs.

4. In a large sauté pan heat 2 tablespoons olive oil. Add the oysters and cook over medium-high heat for 5 minutes. Remove and let cool.
   In the same pan reduce the heat to medium and add another 2 tablespoons of olive oil, the spinach, garlic, salt, and pepper.
   Cook for 8 to 10 minutes until the spinach is wilted.

5. Once the oysters are cool, chop them into small pieces. Divide the oysters among the 8 shells. Top with the wilted spinach. Pour the cream & egg mixture into each shell just up to the top. Top with the breadcrumb mixture and bake for 25 minutes.

Chicken and Sausage Gumbo

A classic New Orleans dish. You will find this on almost every menu at New Orleans restaurants. It's a spicy stew made with meat or shellfish or a combination, served over rice. The word Gumbo comes from the African term for okra (the vegetable used for thickening the stew in some recipes).

Servings: 4-6
Prep time: 15 minutes
Cooking time: 1 hr 45 minutes
Cost: $18.77

Ingredients
4 tablespoons oil
4 tablespoons flour
2 celery stalks, diced
1 yellow onion, diced
1 green bell pepper, diced
½ lb. sausage, sliced into ½ inch slices
1 lb.boneless chicken breast,
    cut into 1 inch cubes
2 x 14.5 oz. cans cut okra
1 x 28 oz. can diced tomatoes
1 x 15.5 oz. can whole kernel corn
1 tablespoon garlic powder
1 teaspoon salt
¼ teaspoon cayenne pepper
3 cups chicken stock
Rice (adjust the amount according to
    the number of guests you are serving)

Equipment
Stock pot (Pasta pot)
Medium saucepan for cooking rice
Measuring cups & spoons

Directions
1. In a stockpot whisk the oil and flour over medium-low heat to create a dark roux—this will take about 3 minutes.

2. Proceed to add the onions, celery, and bell pepper and stir constantly until the vegetables have become tender. This process should take about 5 minutes.

3. Add garlic powder, salt, sausage, cayenne pepper and cook for 2 to 3 minutes. Next add chicken stock, tomatoes, and okra and cook over medium-high heat to bring to a boil. Once the mixture has come to a boil, let it sit uncovered on medium-low heat for 30 minutes. At this point add the cubed chicken and cook uncovered over low heat for 1 hour.

4. While the gumbo is cooking, cook rice in a saucepan according to the package directions.

5. Serve over rice.

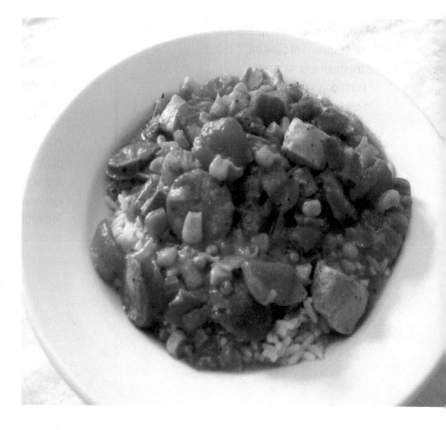

BANANAS FOSTER ICE CREAM

Servings: 6 - 8
Prep time: 5 minutes
Cooking time: 20 minutes
Cost: $4.97

This is our take on a classic New Orleans dish. Created at the famous and fabulous Brennan's restaurant in the French Quarter, the original dish is bananas, brown sugar, cinnamon, rum, and banana liqueur all sautéed together and topped with vanilla ice cream. We've left out the alcohol and combined the traditional ingredients into an original ice cream.

Ingredients
3 ripe bananas, cubed
½ cup brown sugar
4 tablespoons unsalted butter
1 and 2/3 cups heavy cream *
2/3 cup milk *
4 egg yolks
½ cup sugar
1 tsp vanilla extract

Equipment
1 quart ice cream maker
Homemade double boiler—glass bowl and saucepan
1 ½ to 2 quart saucepan
Whisk, wooden spoon, soup ladle
Medium sauté pan

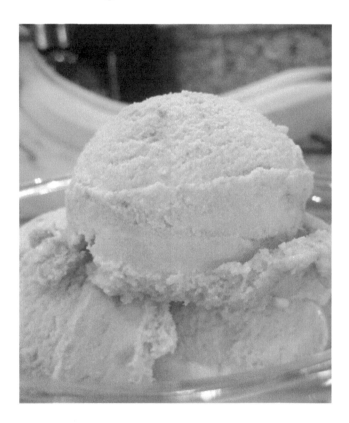

Directions

1. Add the milk, cream, vanilla, and sugar to a saucepan and warm over medium-low heat for 5 to 8 minutes.

2. Whisk the egg yolks in a glass bowl. Meanwhile, make a homemade double boiler: take a 2 quart saucepan, add 2 inches of water and place over medium-high heat until the water boils, then reduce the heat to low. Next, place the glass bowl with the eggs over the saucepan. (See picture in Saffron Ice Cream recipe.) Ladle the warm cream mixture into the eggs slowly in order to temper the eggs. Whisk continuously during this process. (Tempering slowly brings up the temperature of an egg mixture so that the eggs don't scramble.) Cook over low heat until the custard coats the back of a wooden spoon. This will take about 5-8 minutes.

3. In a medium sauté pan, over medium heat, melt the butter and the brown sugar. Stir, then add the banana and stir constantly for about 5 minutes until the sauce thickens and the bananas begin to fall apart. Add the bananas foster to the custard and stir until well combined.

4. Put custard in the refrigerator for 2-3 hours or overnight. Once the custard has cooled add it to your ice cream maker and churn for 30 minutes. This can be eaten directly out of the ice cream maker for a softer version. Transfer to a freezer-safe container and store in the freezer for a firmer version.

Note: You should keep the bowl and blade of your ice cream maker in the freezer so you are always ready to make home-made ice cream.

* This is not a typo; we've adjusted the volume of cream and milk because of the bananas

The Athens Dinner
$9.47 per Person

The menu:
Mezzethes
Moussaka
Rizogalo

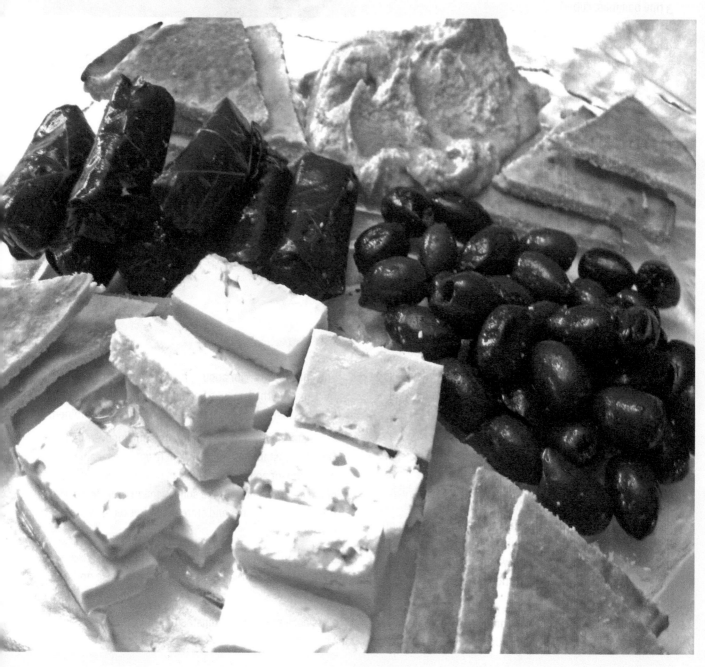

Mezzethes

Mezzethes is a Greek starter plate, similar to Spanish tapas or Italian antipasto. Dolmades, more commonly known as stuffed grape leaves, are very labor intensive to make and readily available in stores. We therefore recommend buying them. You can make the hummus yourself using our recipe from the Finger Foods chapter, or you can buy a store-bought version along with other spreads such as taramosalata (fish egg dip).

Servings: 4
Prep time: 5 minutes
Cooking time: 0 minutes
Cost: $16.96

Ingredients
Dolmades (rice stuffed grape leaves)
Hummus (see our recipe in the Finger Foods chapter)
Feta cheese
Kalamata olives
Pita bread (see our recipe for toasted cumin pita chips in the Finger Foods chapter)

Equipment
None

Directions
Arrange on a platter! Drizzle the feta and the hummus with olive oil.

MOUSSAKA

Moussaka is a classic dish you'll find on every menu throughout Greece. It appears complicated but it is not—but it is time consuming. So make sure you begin cooking 2 hours before your guests are going to arrive. It's loaded with eggplant, ground beef, and smothered in béchamel sauce—so rich and yummie. It's the Greek answer to lasagna.

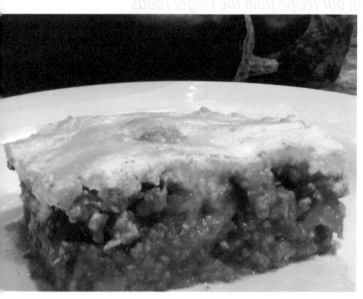

Prep time: 30 minutes
Cooking time: 90 minutes
Servings: 4 - 6
Cost: $18.69

Ingredients

3 eggplants
1 lb. ground beef
1 large or 2 medium yellow onions, chopped
¼ cup olive oil
¼ cup tomato paste
1 tablespoon garlic paste
1 teaspoon salt
½ teaspoon ground black pepper
1 teaspoon ground cinnamon
1 cup grated Parmesan cheese
½ cup bread crumbs
Béchamel sauce (see below)

Béchamel Sauce Ingredients

6 tablespoons butter
6 tablespoons flour
3 cups whole milk
2 eggs
½ teaspoon ground nutmeg

Equipment

Baking sheet or broiler pan
Large sauté pan for ground beef
Large saucepan for béchamel sauce
Mixing bowls
9 x 13 inch baking dish
Measuring cups & spoons

Directions

1. Preheat the oven to broil.

2. Slice the eggplants into ½ inch slices and place on a baking sheet, drizzle with olive oil, and broil for 3 minutes each side. You will need to do this in several batches. Remove from the oven and decrease the oven temperature to 350 degrees F.

3. Meanwhile, in a large sauté pan, sauté the onions with ¼ cup olive oil over medium heat until translucent, about 6 to 8 minutes. Add the meat and brown over medium heat for 10 minutes. Add the tomato paste, garlic, cinnamon, salt and pepper and cook over medium-low for 10 minutes.

For the bechamel sauce:

1. Make a roux by melting 6 tablespoons of butter and add 6 tablespoons of flour over medium-low heat and whisk until a blonde color appears—this takes about 2-3 minutes. Add 3 cups of whole milk slowly, whisking continuously and bring to a boil over medium-high heat then reduce the heat to low, add the nutmeg and cook until thick (8 - 10 minutes).

2. Turn off the heat and cool for 5 minutes then stir in the Parmesan and the eggs.

3. Grease the bottom of the baking dish with 2 tablespoons oil then sprinkle with bread crumbs. Layer the eggplant in the dish, top with the meat mixture, then another layer of eggplant and finish by pouring the Béchamel sauce over the top. Bake for 50 minutes. Let cool for 10 minutes before cutting.

It's great hot or cold!

RIZOGALO (RICE PUDDING)

Ellen grew up eating this for dessert at my Yia-Yia's house. She remembers always going back for seconds. The Greeks love pistachios—you will find them in lots of desserts.

Prep time: 10 minutes
Cooking time: 40 - 45 minutes
Servings: 4
Cost: $2.21

Ingredients

½ cup rice (short grain, Carolina preferably)
¼ teaspoon salt
3 cups milk
¼ cup sugar
½ teaspoon cinnamon
1 teaspoon vanilla extract
¼ cup pistachios (if pistachios are salted, eliminate the salt)

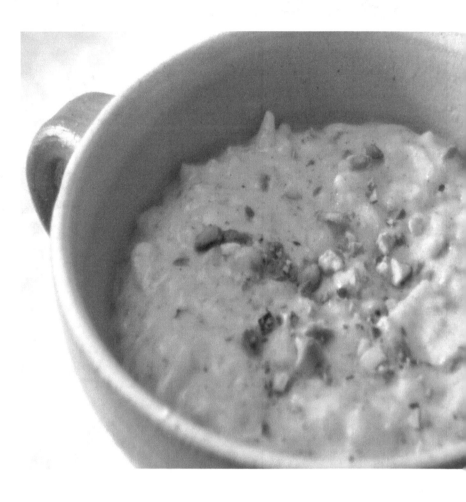

Equipment

Saucepan
Measuring cups
Plastic baggy
Measuring spoons

Directions

1. Cook the rice in 2 ½ cups of milk in a saucepan over low heat for 30 minutes.

2. Place the chopped pistachios in a plastic baggy, then crush with a hard, heavy object (can, mallet, rolling pin, or book) until ground roughly.

3. Once the rice is tender, stir in the remaining ½ cup of milk and bring to a boil, then cook for 1 minute.

4. Add the sugar, half the quantity of pistachios, cinnamon, and vanilla extract. Continue to cook until the pudding has a thick consistency (about 15 – 20 minutes over low heat), then serve in bowls and sprinkle with the remaining pistachio crumbles.

THE SANTA FE DINNER
$9.84 PER PERSON

The menu:
Nachos Extravaganza
Steak Fajitas
Ancho Chile Chocolate Mousse

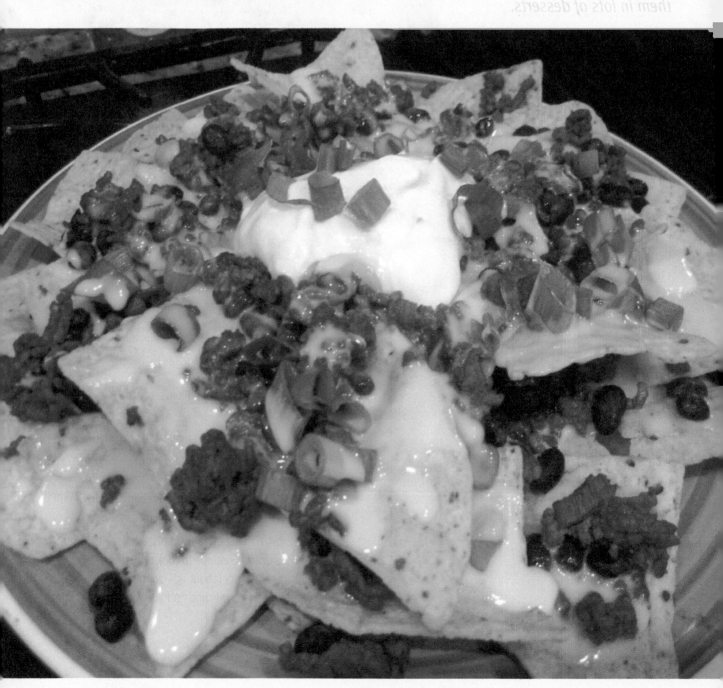

NACHOS EXTRAVAGANZA

Top these nachos with any of your favorite Mexican treats. Add sliced, pickled jalapeno peppers for some added zing!

Prep time: 10 minutes
Cooking time: 25 minutes
Servings: 4
Cost: $14.22

Ingredients

13 oz. package of tortilla chips
1 lb. Queso Blanco cheese (comes in blocks, can be found near the Velveeta)
½ cup milk
1 lb. ground beef
15.5 oz. can of black beans
1 pack taco seasoning mix (comes in 1 to 1.5 ounce packs)
2 green onions (scallions), sliced
Sour cream (optional)

Equipment

Large sauté pan
Medium size microwave safe bowl
2 dinner size plates for serving
Chopping knife

Directions

1. Heat a large sauté pan over medium heat.
   Add 2 tablespoons of olive oil.
   Add the ground beef and cook about 10 minutes—while cooking, chop the meat into small pieces with a spatula.

2. Once the meat is cooked add the taco seasoning mix, ½ cup water, and the beans.
   Let cook over medium-low heat for 10 minutes.

3. For the cheese: Cut the cheese block in cubes and place in a microwave safe bowl.
   Add the milk and microwave for 2 minutes.
   Mix and let sit for 1-2 minutes to thicken.

4. Arrange the chips on 2 dinner size plates.
   Sprinkle meat, beans, and cheese over the chips.
   Repeat for another layer.

5. Top with scallions and sour cream and serve warm.

STEAK FAJITAS

The original fajitas were made with skirt steak and many purists believe that if another cut of meat used it is therefore not a fajita. But the use of the word fajita has changed over time. In most circles it is acceptable to use the terms vegetable fajita, chicken fajita, shrimp fajita. Fajitas are so versatile! You can add your favorite ingredients—the basics are peppers and onions, then a meat or fish, and topped with sour cream, cheese, and salsa—so go wild.

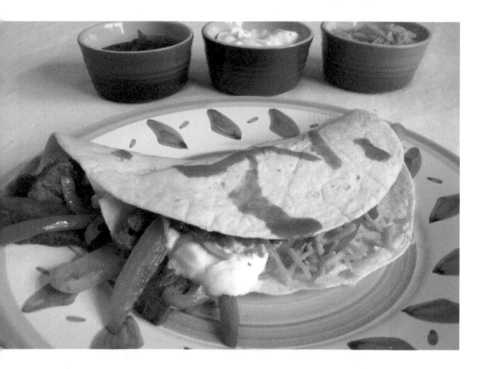

Servings: 4
Prep time: 10 minutes
Cooking time: 30 minutes
Cost: $14.64

Equipment

2 large sauté pans (one for peppers and onions, the other for steak)
Serving bowls for the sour cream, salsa, cheese—or just put a spoon in the jar
Chopping knife

Directions

1. Slice the steak against the grain (cut perpendicular to where you see the direction of the muscle fibers). This can be a tough cut of meat and this will allow it to be very flavorful and tender.

2. Slice the peppers and onion into strips. Heat a large sauté pan over medium-low heat and add the oil, peppers, and onion. Cook for about 20 minutes, until the vegetables are softened.

3. Heat another 2 tablespoons of olive oil in a large sauté pan over medium-high heat. When the pan is hot add the steak, sprinkle with 1teaspoon salt and ½ teaspoon pepper and cook for about 5 to 6 minutes.

4. Take a tortilla and fill with meat, peppers, and top with cheese, salsa, and sour cream. To add heat, add jarred ja lapeños or a couple squirts of your favorite hot sauce. Re member, to cool down heat, milk products work best—so add more sour cream if you've made yours too hot.

Ingredients

1 lb. skirt or skillet steak, sliced into strips
3 bell peppers (yellow, red, green, or a combo), sliced into strips
2 large yellow onions, sliced into strips
8 fajita flour tortillas (2 per person)
1 cup shredded cheddar cheese
1 cup sour cream
1 cup of your favorite salsa
1 teaspoon salt (+ 1 tsp more for sprinkling over meat)
½ teaspoon black pepper (+ ½ tsp more for sprinkling over meat)
Jarred pickled, sliced jalapeños (optional)
Your favorite hot sauce (optional)

ANCHO CHILE CHOCOLATE MOUSSE

This basic recipe for mousse can be easily transformed to satisfy any taste desires. Leave out the chile powder and you have rich chocolate mousse. Experiment with different chocolates for a different flavors and richness. And experiment with different glasses for presentation. Half the fun of cooking is presenting your final product.

Servings: 4
Prep time: 10 minutes
Cooking time: 5 minutes
Cost: $8.50

Ingredients
4 oz. dark chocolate, chopped
4 oz. milk chocolate, chopped
10 oz. heavy cream
1 tablespoon Ancho Chile powder
4 egg whites, beaten to soft peaks
1/3 cup sugar
4 oz. heavy cream, extra

Equipment
Food processor
Electronic hand mixer (strongly recommended but not required)
Large mixing bowls
Small saucepan
Glasses for serving

Directions
Prepare the day before cooking!

1. In a food processor, blend the chocolate until grated. If you have a mini-food processor, you will need to do this process in several stages. Heat a small saucepan over medium heat and warm the cream to a scalding temperature, just under boiling (less than 5 minutes). Once the cream has heated, add it little by little to the food processor and blend until the chocolate is completely smooth.

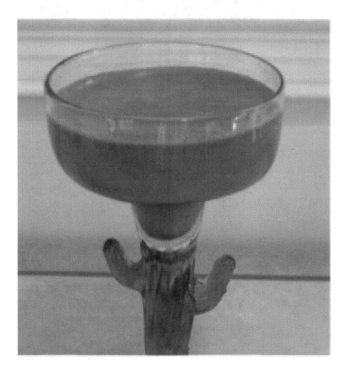

2. If you do not own hand beater (which can be purchased for as low as $20), you can beat the egg whites with a whisk by hand. It's great exercise for your arm and takes about 15 minutes of diligent beating, until the whites form into stiff peaks. *

3. In a separate bowl, whip the extra heavy cream until a soft peak is formed.

4. Pour the chocolate into a large mixing bowl and then fold the beaten egg whites into the chocolate, carefully turning until the two have combined completely. Then fold in the whipped extra heavy cream. This must now be chilled before serving.

   You have 2 options: (1) leave in a large mixing bowl to chill and when the mousse is ready you can scoop servings from this bowl, (2) pour unset mousse into serving glasses and then chill. Chill in the fridge for at least 3 hours or overnight.

Alternative preparation option:
You can buy chocolate chips or flakes if you want to skip the food processor step. In this case, the hot cream will melt the chips or flakes for you.

* stiff peaks = the peak stands straight up
* soft peaks = the peak bends over

...mpanied to satisfy any taste desires.

...eave out the chile powder and you have

...milk chocolate mousse. Experiment with

...different chocolates for a different flavors

...and richness. And experiment with differ-

...ent glasses for presentation. Half the fun

...of cooking is presenting your final product.

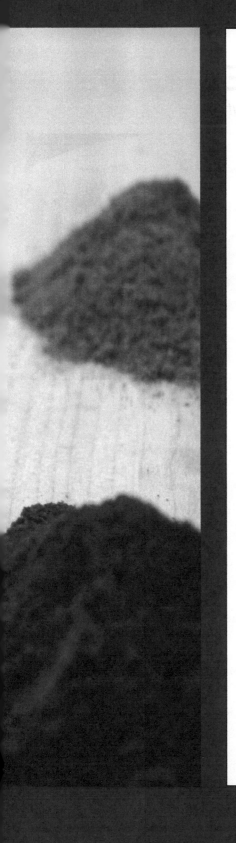

Lyon, $11.43 per person

Siena, $11.73 per person

South Beach, $12.22 per person

Bar Harbor, $14.07 per person

LYON, FRANCE DINNER
$11.43 PER PERSON

The menu:
Salad Lyonnaise, Beef Wellington with Béarnaise Sauce, Cheese Course, Chocolate Truffles

SALAD LYONNAISE

This is a traditional salad you will find everywhere in France but particularly in Lyon. It's a meal at lunchtime.

Servings: 4
Prep Time: 5 minutes
Cooking Time: 20 minutes
Cost: $6.88

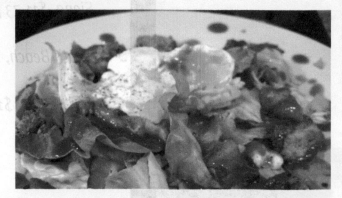

Salad Ingredients

12 slices bacon (½ pound)
4 large eggs, poached
Frisee (or salad mix with frisee in it)
3 slices honey wheat bread, ½ inch thick
1 tablespoon bacon grease
1 tablespoon champagne vinegar

Dijon vinaigrette ingredients

1 teaspoon Dijon mustard
2 tablespoons red wine vinegar
6 tablespoons olive oil
½ teaspoon salt
¼ teaspoon pepper

Equipment

Sauté pan (can be used for both the bacon
    and the croutons)
Medium saucepan
Small mixing bowl
Slotted spoon
Whisk

Directions

1. Cook the bacon in a sauté pan over medium heat until crispy. Reserve about 1 tablespoon of oil from the bacon to cook the croutons.
2. Slice the bacon into 1 inch bite-sized pieces, using three slices per plate. Add to the bed of greens.

Cut the bread into cubes the size of croutons. Heat the oil in the sauté pan over medium-high, then add the croutons and let sauté for about 2 minutes. Stir occasionally to make sure all sides have been lightly toasted. Sprinkle with salt and pepper.

To poach the eggs:
Bring 2 inches of water in a medium saucepan to a slow simmer (slow boil). To do this bring the water to a bowl over high heat then turn down the heat to medium-low. Add 1 tablespoon of champagne vinegar. Gently crack each egg into separate prep bowls, then pour into the simmering liquid. Be careful not to break the yolk! Allow the egg to cook undisturbed for 3 minutes. Use a slotted spoon to remove and gently place on the bed of greens.

To make the vinaigrette:
Whisk the Dijon mustard, vinegar, salt and pepper together in a small mixing bowl. Add the olive oil in a slow stream and whisk until thoroughly blended.

To make the finished salad:
Place the poached egg in the middle of the greens, sprinkle with croutons, lardons (bacon), and dressing. Break the egg yolk and mix in with the salad—this adds incredible flavor to the dressing and makes it an authentic salad you would find at a café in Lyon.

BEEF WELLINGTON WITH BÉARNAISE SAUCE

This is perhaps the easiest beef wellington recipe you'll find anywhere. Ellen was inspired by her in-laws, JoAnne Pappano and Robert Norton. They serve this every Christmas and stuff the pastry with either sautéed mushrooms or liver paté. Just place your ingredients down on the puff pastry then top with meat then fold the pastry over the meat. Really easy and really yummie!

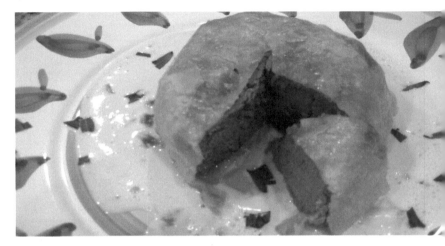

Servings: 4
Prep time: 15 minutes
Cooking time: 25 minutes
Cost: $22.10

Béarnaise Sauce Ingredients
2 tablespoons chopped fresh tarragon
¼ cup champagne vinegar
2 tablespoons diced shallot
3 egg yolks + 1 egg for egg wash
1 stick butter, melted

Filet Wellington Ingredients
4 pieces filet mignon (about 4 ounces each)
1 sheet puff pastry (remove from freezer and thaw 1 hour before baking)
All purpose flour for rolling out pastry
 (about 2 tablespoons)
Salt and pepper to season the meat

Equipment
Baking sheet
Blender
Saucepan
Pastry brush (optional)
Parchment paper (optional, for easy cleanup)

Directions
Preheat the oven to 400 degrees F.

To start the béarnaise sauce:
1. Combine the diced shallots, finely chopped tarragon, champagne vinegar, a pinch of salt, and a pinch of pepper in a small saucepan.
2. Cook at medium heat until the liquid is reduced to about 2 tablespoons (approximately 3 – 5 minutes). Be sure to watch carefully!

For the wellington:
1. Roll out one puff pastry sheet and cut into 4 squares.
2. Stretch the pastry over the filet, covering all sides and sealing. Place the filet seam side down on the baking sheet over parchment paper.
3. Using either a pastry brush or a spoon, brush the puff pastry with an egg wash (an egg wash is 1 egg mixed with either 1 teaspoon of milk, cream or water).
4. Cook for 25 minutes at 400 degrees for medium-rare steaks.

If you want to sear your steaks first, sear over medium-high heat, searing each side of the steak (about 5 minutes total), then place on the puff pastry sheet and cook for 18 minutes for medium-rare steaks.

To finish the béarnaise sauce:
1. Blend the tarragon mix and 3 egg yolks in a blender.
2. Heat 1 stick of salted butter in a saucepan over medium-low heat until melted or place in the microwave for 1 minute (you can rinse and use the same saucepan you did for the tarragon mixture).
3. With the blender running, add the hot butter in a slow drizzle.
4. Once the wellingtons have finished cooking, set each one on a plate and add generous amounts of Béarnaise sauce.

And there you have it, Filet Wellington with Béarnaise!

CHEESE COURSE

The cheese course is served after dinner in France.
Most French eat the cheese course without bread or crackers.
Crackers are perfect for cleansing the palate in between cheeses,
so we recommend keeping them on hand while dining.

Ingredients

1 chunk hard cheese
    (cheddar, gouda, Norwegian goat)
1 chunk goat cheese
1 chunk creamy cheese
    (brie, camembert, triple cream, St. Andre)
1 chunk of something different
    (Spanish Manchego, French Chaumes)

Arrange the cheese on a platter with crackers or baguette slices.

You'll probably have leftover cheese. You can make cheese omelets or grilled cheese sandwiches with the leftovers.

Servings: 4 +
Prep time: 5 minutes
Cooking time: 0
Cost: $15.00

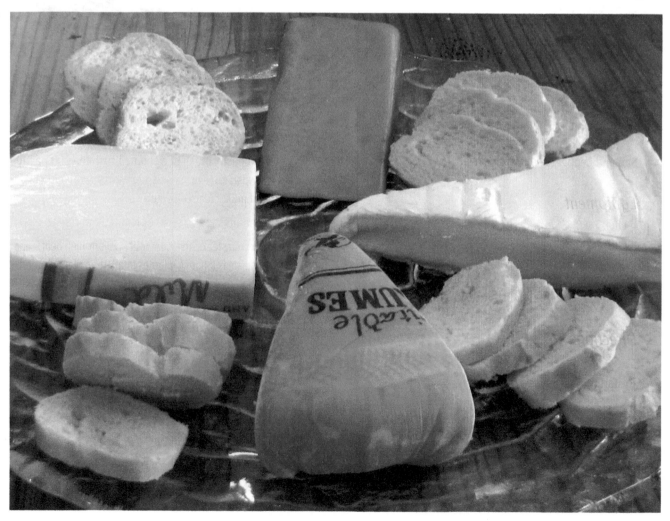

CHOCOLATE TRUFFLES

Easy, easy, easy! This French meal might seem intimidating at first but you'll marvel at the ease and taste. Dust your truffles in crushed nuts or powdered sugar if you wish.

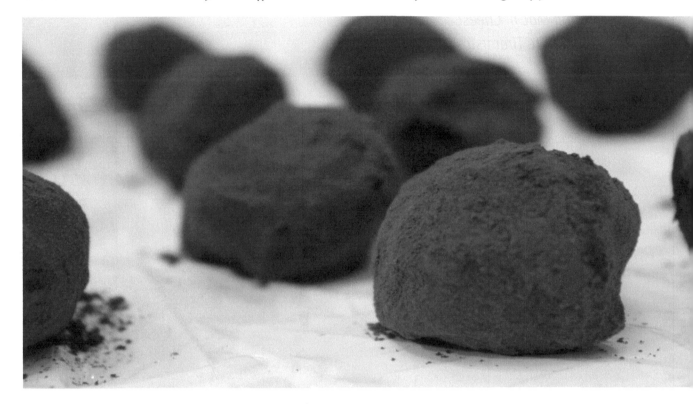

Servings: makes 20 truffles
Prep time: 20 minutes
Cooking time: 5 minutes
Cooling time: 1 hour
Cost: $1.72

Ingredients
8 oz. bittersweet chocolate
4 oz. (1/2 cup) cream
Powdered cocoa (optional)

Equipment
Saucepan
Whisk
Small ice cream scoop

Directions

1. In a small saucepan, heat the cream to just below a bowl over medium heat.

2. Lower the heat to medium-low. Add the chocolate to the sauce pan and mix until blended and smooth. The chocolate should take on a shiny, smooth consistency.

3. Allow it to cool in the fridge for 10 minutes, then remove and whisk vigorously with a wire whisk for 1 full minute. Cover and chill for 1 hour.

4. After the chocolate has cooled, scoop out with a small ice cream scoop onto parchment paper. Roll the chocolate into balls. Be sure to have a cup of hot water on hand to dip the scooper into.

5. When you are ready to serve, have a bowl with cocoa powder on hand nearby. Roll the truffles gently between your palms to attain a rounder shape, cover them with cocoa powder and place on a plate.

Fresh truffles can be kept in the fridge for two weeks!

Good truffles are all about the quality of chocolate you use—the higher the quality, the better the truffles.

THE SIENA DINNER
$11.73 PER PERSON

The menu:
Artichokes with Lemon-Lime Aioli
Saffron Mac n' Cheese
Ten-Minute Tiramisu

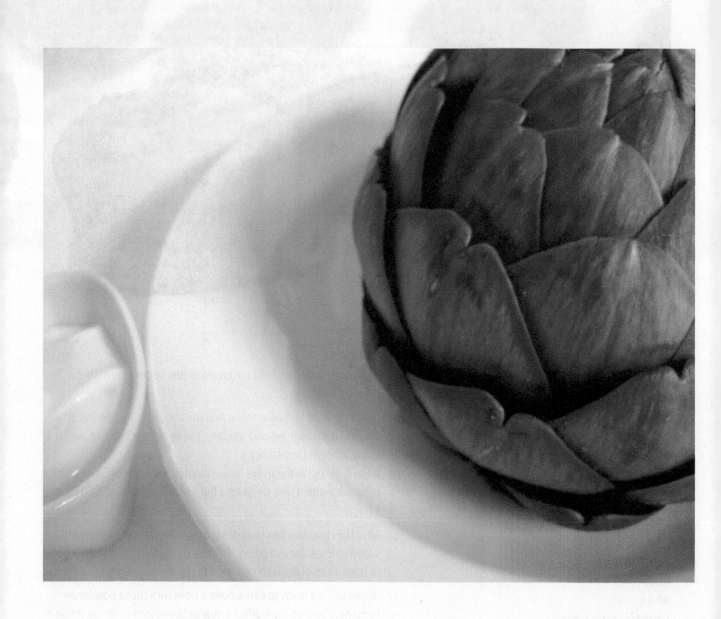

ARTICHOKES WITH LEMON-LIME AIOLI

Don't eat the whole leaf (don't laugh, I had a friend do this once). Just the end part with the meat—hold it by the spiny end and slide your teeth over the meaty opposite end. It's delicious dipped in butter too. Or if you're watching your calories don't dip at all—artichokes are very low in calories.

Ingredients

4 medium or large artichokes
1 teaspoon salt
1 teaspoon garlic powder
1 teaspoon onion powder
Aioli
1 cup mayonnaise
1 tablespoon lemon juice
1 tablespoon lime juice

Servings: 4
Prep time: 5 minutes
Cooking time: 1 hour
Cost: $6.44

Equipment

Large stockpot
Mixing bowl

Directions

1. Place 2 inches of water in a large stockpot and bring to a boil over high heat.

2. Add the salt, garlic powder, onion powder, and artichokes and reduce the heat to medium-low, cover and cook for about 1 hour. The artichoke is done when you can easily pull a leaf off.

3. In a mixing bowl, mix the mayonnaise with the lemon and lime juices and separate into 4 small bowls. Each person will have his or her own aioli dipping sauce.

SAFFRON MAC N' CHEESE

This is definitely not your average mac n' cheese. The saffron adds such an interesting flavor and with Japanese bread crumbs (Panko) on top, you've got an instant elegant dish for your dinner party. You can serve it with a side salad but it can easily stand alone. Don't forget you're starting the meal with artichokes so you get your greens in the first course. Serves 6 as a main course.

Servings: 4 - 6
Prep time: 10 minutes
Cooking time: 45 minutes
Cost: $14.71

Ingredients
1 lb. box of shells
4 cups sharp cheddar cheese (2 x 8 ounce packages of shredded cheese)
½ cup mascarpone cheese (usually found in the gourmet cheese section)
¼ cup Parmesan cheese
3 cups milk
2 tablespoons butter (+ extra for buttering baking dish)
2 tablespoons flour
1 teaspoon saffron threads
1 teaspoon salt
½ teaspoon black pepper
½ teaspoon ground nutmeg
Crumb topping:
1 ½ cups bread crumbs, preferably Panko
4 tablespoons butter, melted

Equipment
Stock pot
Large saucepan
9 x 13 baking dish
Microwave-safe mixing bowl

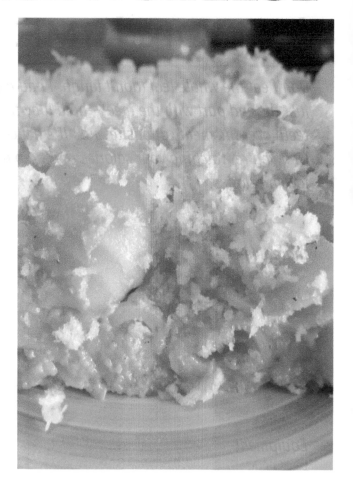

Directions

1. Preheat the oven to 375 degrees F.

2. Cook the pasta according to the package directions, drain and set aside.

3. For the topping, melt the butter in the microwave for about 20 seconds. Mix with the Panko and set aside.

4. For the sauce, melt the butter in a large saucepan, add the flour and whisk until you have a blonde roux. Add the milk slowly and turn up the heat to medium-high for about 1-2 minutes until the mixture begins to boil. Turn down the heat to medium-low and add the saffron, salt, pepper, and nutmeg. Cook for about 10-12 minutes until the mixture begins to thicken.

5. Turn off the heat, add the cheeses and pour over the cooked pasta. Put the pasta in the baking dish and sprinkle with the breadcrumb topping.

6. Bake for 18-20 minutes, until bubbling. Let stand for 10 minutes, and serve.

Ten-Minute Tiramisu

Yes, tiramisu in 10 minutes. You'll find scores of tiramisu recipes out there but ours is the quickest and most delicious.

Ingredients

16 oz. of mascarpone cheese (leave on counter for
    1 hour to soften)
1 cup powdered sugar
½ cup unsweetened cocoa powder
1 teaspoon vanilla
1 cup coffee
1 tablespoon sugar (granulated or powdered)
2 packages ladyfingers (we prefer soft for this recipe)
Chocolate covered espresso beans for garnish

Equipment

Large mixing bowl
Hand mixer
Pie dish or 9 x 9 baking dish (for dipping lady fingers)
Measuring cups & spoons
Martini glasses for serving

Directions

1. Pour hot coffee into the pie dish and add 1 tablespoon of sugar and mix.

2. In a large mixing bowl mix the mascarpone, 1 cup powdered sugar, cocoa, and vanilla with a hand mixer for 2 minutes until smooth.

3. Get your glasses ready. Dip each ladyfinger in the coffee for only a second—you don't want your ladyfingers to get soggy. Place 2 ladyfingers in the bottom of the martini glass and press down. Cover with a heaping tablespoon of mascarpone, top with another layer of coffee soaked ladyfingers, then another layer of mascarpone, one more layer of ladyfingers and finish with mascarpone.

4. Sprinkle with chocolate covered espresso beans. It tastes best when refrigerated for at least 2 hours (you can also eat it immediately if you can't wait—we do!).

5. You can make the tiramisu 2 days in advance of your party. The martini glasses take up a lot of room in the refrigerator so if you wish you can use a 9 x 9 baking dish and layer as above and refrigerate.

Serve like lasagna.

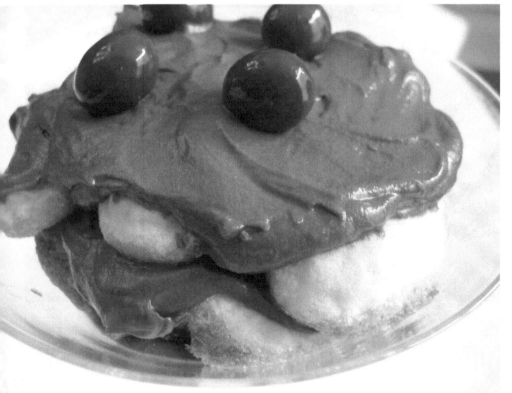

Servings: 4
Prep time: 10 minutes
Cooking time: 0 minutes
Cost: $14.03

SOUTH BEACH DINNER
$12.22 PER PERSON

The menu:
Heirloom Caprese Salad
Mahi-Mahi with Lime Cilantro Salsa
Coconut Lime Macaroons

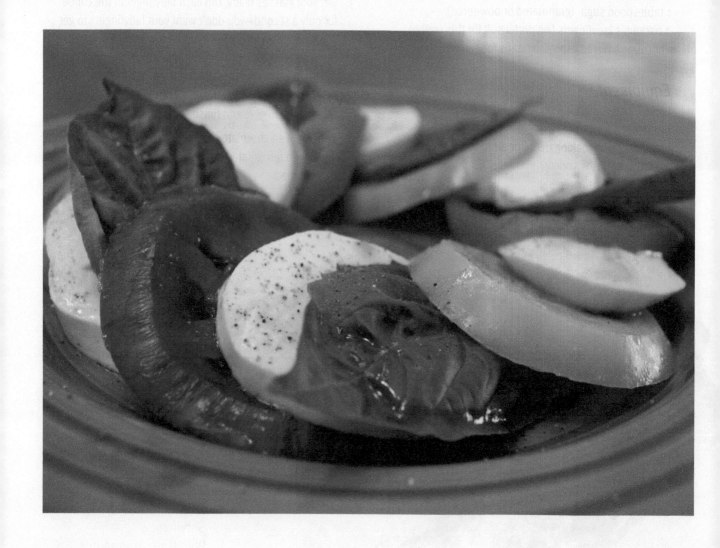

HEIRLOOM CAPRESE SALAD

A lot of debate surrounds the definition of a true heirloom tomato—50-year-old seed? 100-year-old seed? Open pollination? Unless you want to be a tomato aficionado then frankly who cares—the bottom line is that heirloom tomatoes are perhaps the sweetest, richest, most flavorful tomato you will ever eat.

Servings: 4
Prep time: 10 minutes
Cooking time: 0 minutes
Cost: $ 20.00

Ingredients

3 heirloom tomatoes
    (select different colors if available)
8 fresh basil leaves
2 balls fresh mozzarella
4 tablespoons olive oil
4 pinches of salt
4 pinches of pepper

Equipment

Cutting board
Serrated knife for slicing tomatoes

Directions

1. On a cutting board, using a serrated knife, slice the heirloom tomatoes into ½ inch thick slices.

2. Slice the fresh mozzarella the same way, then arrange on a plate.

3. Sprinkle with ground black pepper, salt, and drizzle with olive oil.

4. Add some basil leaves on the sides or the top to add garnish (and a delicious contrast to the juicy flavors of the cheese and tomatoes).

MAHI-MAHI WITH LIME CILANTRO SALSA

Mahi-mahi is also known as dolphin-fish or Dorado. Do not confuse this fish with a dolphin, which is a mammal. This meal is all about what South Beach is all about—light, elegant, flavorful food with a Caribbean flare.

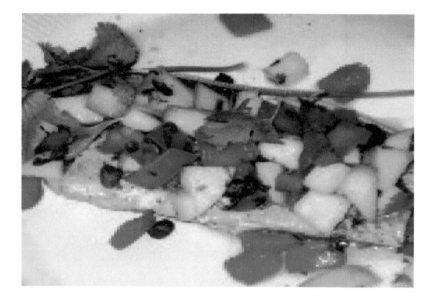

Servings: 4
Prep time: 10 minutes
Cooking time: 10 minutes
Cost: $19.74

Ingredients
2 lb. fresh mahi-mahi (6 – 8 oz per person)
2 tablespoons vegetable oil
1 granny smith apple, diced
1 red pepper, diced
2 tablespoons capers
¼ cup lime juice
2 tablespoons cilantro, chopped
1 teaspoon salt
½ teaspoon ground black pepper

Equipment
Large sauté pan
Cutting board
Chopping knife/paring knife

Directions
1. To make the salsa, chop pepper, apple, and cilantro and toss with capers, limejuice, salt and pepper.

2. Season the mahi-mahi on both sides with salt and pepper.

3. Preheat a large sauté pan on medium and add 2 tablespoons of vegetable oil.

4. Cook the mahi-mahi about 4-5 minutes per side. The fish should be opaque, and a knife should slide in easily.

COCONUT LIME MACAROONS

Two New Englanders' answer to the key lime pie—macaroons with a Floridian twist. Yet another dish you'll start to have cravings for. I think I'm having one right now!

Servings: 4
Prep time: 10 minutes
Cooking time: 25 minutes
Cost: $9.13

Ingredients

3 cups shredded sweetened coconut flakes
14 oz. sweetened condensed milk (1 can)
2 egg whites, beaten until they form stiff white peaks
6 tablespoons lime juice
2 teaspoons vanilla extract
¼ teaspoon salt
Zest of 1 lime

Equipment

Mixing bowls
Whisk or electric hand mixer
Cooking sheet
Parchment paper (optional)

Directions

1. Preheat the oven to 325 degrees F.

2. Mix the coconut, condensed milk, lime, vanilla, and salt in a large mixing bowl.

3. In a separate bowl beat the egg whites until they form stiff peaks (this can be done by hand with a whisk or with an electric mixer with the whisk attachment).

4. Gently mix (fold) the egg whites into the coconut mixture.

5. Place a tablespoon amount on a baking sheet and bake for 25 minutes.

6. Sprinkle with lime zest immediately when they come out of the oven.

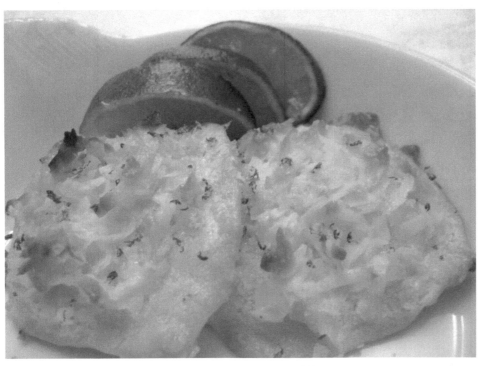

THE BAR HARBOR DINNER
$14.07 PER PERSON

The menu:
Fried Oysters
Blue Lobster Burger
Apple Blueberry Crumb Pie

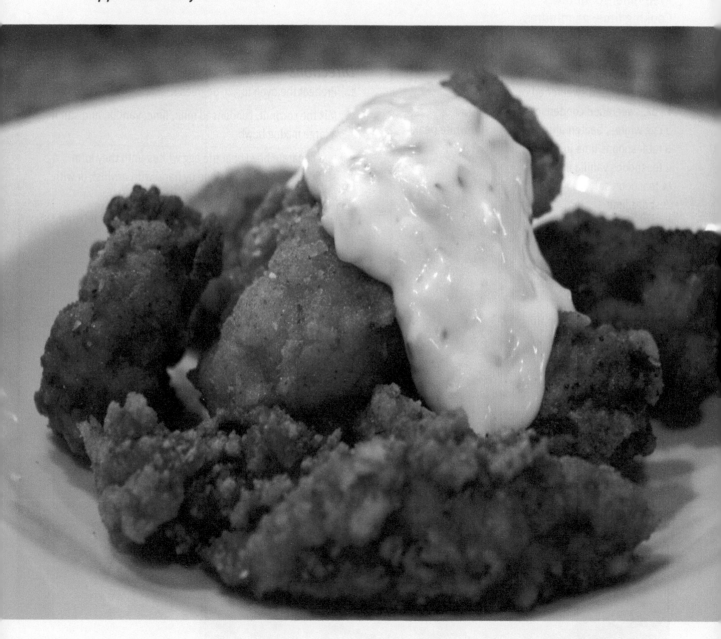

FRIED OYSTERS

These are great alone or on a sandwich. You'll feel like you are at the shore watching the waves and seagulls.

Servings: 4
Prep time: 10 minutes
Cooking time: 15 minutes
Cost: $24.31

Ingredients

1 pound fresh oysters (comes in 8 oz plastic containers in most stores)
2 cups of fish fry (bread crumb/corn flour mixture available in most supermarkets, you will find it near the fish)
1 cup buttermilk
10 squirts of your favorite hot sauce
Vegetable oil for frying—never have the oil more than half way up the pan

Tartar sauce ingredients

3 heaping tablespoons of mayonnaise
2 heaping teaspoons of sweet relish
1 teaspoon of lemon juice
1/8 teaspoon cayenne pepper

Equipment

Large saucepan, 4 inches deep
Strainer for draining oysters
2 mixing bowls
   (one for buttermilk and the other for fish fry)
Small mixing bowl for tartar sauce

Directions for frying the oysters

1. Fill the saucepan with oil—half way up only.

2. Heat the oil over medium heat for about 5 minutes—the temperature should be 350 degrees.
   If you have a candy thermometer you can place it in the oil and leave it there to monitor your temperature.
   For best results invest in the candy thermometer so you can monitor your temperature.

3. In a mixing bowl add together the buttermilk and hot sauce.

4. Pour the fish fry mixture into another bowl.

5. Line up the bowls next to the stove.

6. Drain the oysters.

7. Dip the oysters in the buttermilk then into the fish fry and slowly place (do not drop) the oysters into the hot oil. Turn the oysters once with tongs. Do not overcrowd the pan with oysters—the temperature of the oil will drop and they will not cook properly and be very greasy.
   It should take about 4 minutes to cook each batch of oysters. You will need to cook 3 to 4 batches depending on the size of your pan.
   Make sure your oil is at 350 degrees F for each batch.

8. Remove them and place on a paper towel to drain excess oil. Sprinkle with salt and serve with tartar sauce.

To make the tartar sauce:

1. Mix together all of the ingredients. Homemade tartar sauce is light and refreshing.

2. To serve, place oysters on a small dish and add a dollop of tartar sauce on top.

BLUE LOBSTER BURGER

Surf and turf on a sandwich. Serve coleslaw on the side—or pile it high on the sandwich.

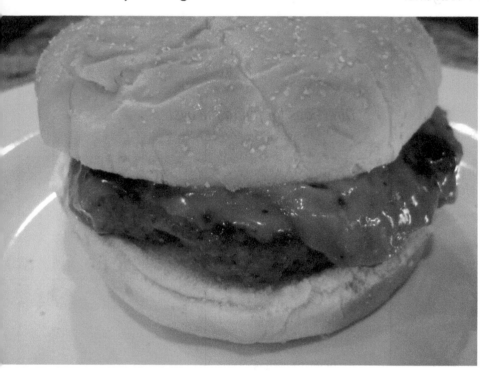

Servings: 6
Prep time: 10 minutes
Cook time: 10-12 minutes
Cost: $21.54

Ingredients

1 lb. ground beef
1 cup cooked lobster meat *
½ cup heavy cream
1 heaping tablespoon blueberry preserves
2 tablespoons unsalted butter
1 teaspoon salt
½ teaspoon black pepper

Aioli ingredients

4 tablespoons mayonnaise
2 heaping tablespoons blueberry preserves
1 tablespoon lemon juice
1 teaspoon lime juice

Equipment

Sauté pan
Saucepan (for boiling lobster tails)
2 mixing bowls
Measuring cups & spoons

Directions

1. If you purchased raw lobster tails, thaw them in the fridge for 3 to 4 hours, then place in boiling water for 10 minutes. Let cool, remove the shell and cut into small chunks.

2. To make the burgers, mix together the beef, lobster, cream, blueberry preserves, salt and pepper. Form into 6 individual burgers.

3. Heat a large sauté pan over medium heat, melt the butter, and cook the burgers for 6 minutes on each side (until well-done).

For the aioli:
Mix the aioli ingredients together. Spread on the top and bottom buns for a juicy burger.

* Lobster can be purchased in a supermarket, fish store, or on the Internet. The most readily available form is frozen lobster tails that come in packages of two (5-6 ounces = enough to make 1 cup cooked meat). It is also available in cans. This lobster meat is knuckle and claw meat and is cooked.

APPLE BLUEBERRY CRUMB PIE

A New England favorite. Especially in the land of blueberries—Maine. The best apples for making apple pie are Jonagold, Jonathan, Granny Smith, and Pippin. The worst are Red Delicious, Gala, Fuji, McIntosh, and Cortland. You can mix apple types also. McIntosh and Cortland are delicious apples in a pie but the problem is that they become mushy when cooked.

Servings: 8
Prep time: 20 minutes
Cooking time: 50 minutes
Cost: $8.52

Ingredients for the pie
1 premade frozen deepdish 9" piecrust
4 – 5 apples
4 tablespoons blueberry preserves
2 tablespoons flour
2 tablespoons lemon juice
½ teaspoon cinnamon
1/8 teaspoon nutmeg
1/8 teaspoon salt

Ingredients for the crumb topping
½ cup flour
½ cup oats
½ cup brown sugar
6 tablespoons melted unsalted butter
¼ cup baker's coconut
½ teaspoon vanilla
½ teaspoon cinnamon

Equipment
Mixing bowls
Measuring cups & spoons
Knife
Baking sheet (optional)

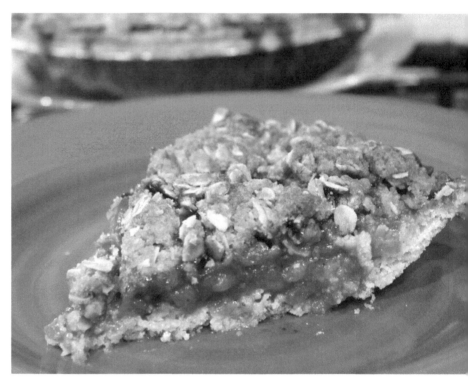

Directions
1. Preheat the oven to 375 degrees F.

2. Cut and core the apples and slice thinly. Put the apples in a large mixing bowl and add blueberry preserves, flour, lemon juice, cinnamon, nutmeg, and salt.

3. Use the piecrust according to the package directions—most can be used right out of the freezer. Pour the apple mixture into the crust.

4. For the crumb topping:
   Mix together all the ingredients and sprinkle over the pie, spreading evenly.

5. Bake at 375 degrees for 60 minutes.

6. Let cool for 20 to 30 minutes. Enjoy with some homemade ice cream; try it with our saffron ice cream.

APPLE BLUEBERRY CRUMB PIE

A New England favorite. Especially in the land of blueberries—Maine. The best apples for making apple pie are Greening, Jonathan, Granny Smith, and Pippin. The worst are Red Delicious, Gala, Fuji, McIntosh, and Cortland. You can mix apple types also. McIntosh and Cortland are delicious apples in a pie but the problem is that they become mushy when cooked.

Ingredients for the

Ingredients for the
crumb topping

Directions

Equipment